I HAVE A CHOICE?!

Bera Dordoni, N.D.

*A Reader-Friendly Introduction to
Building and Strengthening
the Immune System*

Edited by
Claudia Suzanne

The health suggestions in this book are based on the training, personal experiences, and research of the author. Each person is unique and each set of circumstances is unique. Therefore, the author, editor and publisher urge the reader to check with a qualified health professional before using any procedure where there is any question as to its appropriateness.

The author and publisher do not advocate the use of any particular diet or procedure, but believe that the information presented in this book should be available to the public. Always consult with your health-care provider before beginning any new health program.

Because there is always some risk involved, the author and publisher are not responsible for any adverse effects or consequences resulting from the use of any of the suggestions, preparations, or procedures in this book. Please do not use the book if you are unwilling to assume the risk. Feel free to consult a qualified health professional. It is a sign of wisdom, not cowardice, to seek a second or third opinion.

This book is dedicated to those who never knew they had the option to make their own choices, but who choose to do so now.

Copyright © 1995 - Published in 1995 by B.F. Publishing, a division of The Beron Foundation

All rights reserved. No part of this publication may be reproduced, stored in a retrieval system, or transmitted, in any form or by any means, electronic, mechanical, photocopying, recording, or otherwise, without the prior written permission of the copyright owner.

Cover design: Nancy Fischbeck
Editor: Claudia Suzanne
Illustrations: Courtesy of RCD Graphics Group
Printer: B.F. Publishing

Library of Congress Cataloging-in-Publications Data

Dordoni, Bera
   I Have A Choice?!
   Includes Reference section

ISBN 0-9645609-6-8

B.F. Publishing
P.O. Box 2712-344
Huntington Beach, CA 92647
1 (800) 544-7264

Printed in the United States of America

Acknowledgments

Mario, my angel, this book is for you.......

One day when I was asked to write about alternative forms of treatment that could be used for AIDS and cancer patients, as well as others with debilitating dis-eases, I wrote a treatise that I had trouble re-reading. BORING, was all I could think about it. How...how to write something of interest as an introduction to building and strengthening the immune system? While talking with one of my greatest teachers, Jim Ballinger, he encouraged me to write about one or more of my patients' experiences so everyone would be able to relate to the information on a human-interest level. Hence, Tom DoRight was born. Thank you, Jim Ballinger, for being one of the greatest lights in my life.

I'd be nowhere without the incredible assistance I received from my editor, Claudia Suzanne. Her superior skill, sense of humor and keep-to-it-iveness helped make this book what it is today.

Several people let me know when they thought I wasn't clear enough, and I thank them for focusing me...my mom and dad, whose knowledge is so great and whose support made this project possible; my sister Beth for her constructive and humorous critique; my precious friend Mario for asking for recipes so he would know what to do with the foods suggested. Nancy, thank you for the beautiful cover--what communication. Katie, I thank you for your proofreading skills; and Ron, thank you for believing in me always, never letting me quit, and always encouraging me to share with others. I love you all.

Author's Preface

I HAVE A CHOICE?! is an introduction to building and strengthening the human immune system. We all have different options available to each of us when it comes to our personal health care. Once victims, none of us need be victimized again. We do have a choice!

Debilitating diseases such as AIDS, cancer, heart disease and multiple sclerosis are common, everyday occurrences that were not so common 50 years ago. Why? Our modern-day society has brought us to the point where most of our lives are being lived on the run. Stress runs rampant, fear rules the streets, and most people are hustling just to survive in the present economy. We have no time to take care of ourselves--we're in too much of a hurry. Consequently, our immune systems break down, and we end up "getting" any one of the above-named diseases--or some other ailment with a slightly different name or different set of symptoms.

Rather than take the time to correct the circumstances that led to our immune-system breakdown, most of us run to our doctors, demanding a prescription for immediate symptomatic relief. Or check through our drugstore shelves for over-the-counter symptom supressors. We don't recognize that these symptoms are the end result of our lifestyles.

This book is about a gentleman named Tom--but it could be about you, or someone you know. It contains information about healing foods, destructive foods, the joy of juicing, green grasses, herbs, homeopathy, antioxidants, body maintenance, eliminating arthritis from the body, attitude and more.

This book does not take the place of consulting with a health practitioner. It merely offers information on general, non-invasive immune-sytem building and disease recovery. *I Have A Choice?!* presents a different perspective on health care and self-awareness, and invites the reader to explore the concepts of alternative preventative measures and recovery treatments.

CONTENTS

1.	Always In Control	1
2.	Warning Signs	4
3.	The Crisis	10
4.	The Choice	15
5.	What Did I Do?	25
6.	Back To School	31
7.	The State Of Dis-Ease	44
8.	Body Maintenance	48
9.	Vital Energy	57
10.	Lifestyle Adjustments	60
11.	Premium Fuel	68
12.	Mix and Match	74
13.	Proper Food Combining	81
14.	The Group	90
15.	Healing Foods	96
16.	Destructive Foods	111
17.	Liquids & Juicing	119
18.	Grasses & Cleansing	132
19.	Homeopathy	141
20.	A Key Element In Healing	153

...Contents

21.	Antioxidants	155
22.	Herbs & Mushrooms	164
23.	Hydrogen Peroxide	171
24.	Arthritis	175

Choices We Made (Author & Editor)
    Bera's Story   182
    Claudia's Story   187
Keys to a Healthy Life   190
References   194

1 - ALWAYS IN CONTROL

Everyone liked and respected Tom DoRight, the famous director. He always had the perfect answer and a glowing smile for anyone who could capture his attention. He was the biggest moneymaker to come along since Spielberg, and his office shelves--crammed with his many awards--and his waiting room walls--filled with plaques, testimonials and citations--proved it.

Tom only worked with the best in the field--no matter what the field was. His sound men were geniuses, his lighting people were whizzes. His special-effects contracts went to the most sought-after company in the business. Top composers fought for the chance to score his films. Besides keeping the best west coast entertainment lawyer on retainer, he always had an expert business lawyer keeping tab on his many investments, and a top-of-the-line tax attorney to keep the IRS off his back.

Yes, specialists were the only way to go. They kept him on top and in control--not only of all of his projects, but of his life. Control was power.

Tom liked power.

Tom's latest project was a movie-of-the-week. Of course, he always stressed out when he worked on television scripts--the censorship was so stifling to his creativity. Nevertheless, he knew he had to stay liquid--had to keep up with those multiple mortgages--so he lived with the stress.

Fortunately, Tom's crew cooperated on every level to make his life easy on the set. His personal assistant made sure he had piping hot coffee every morning as soon as he got to the set--2 creams, 2 sugars. He could count on finding a soda at hand whenever he wanted one. An aide appeared to light his cigarette every time he pulled one out of the pack, and another would fetch a hamburger and seasoned fries with all the fixings for him as soon as he looked hungry. Yes, Tom DoRight was treated like a king--the only problem was, the king had a constant stomachache. He decided to see his friend, Dr. Don Belcher, a specialist in gastrointestinal disorders.

Tom had known Don Belcher since high school, and had never lost touch with him. When Don graduated at the top of his med-school class, Tom knew he was destined to be one of the best in his field. Over the years, he had risen to be Chief of Staff at the most prestigious hospital in Los Angeles.

Don would know just the right kind of pill to put Tom back on his feet immediately.

2 - WARNING SIGNS

"Hey, Tommy, how ya doing?" Dr. Belcher asked his friend. "Not so good, Donny, my stomach's killing me. I've taken Mylanta, but that doesn't help anymore. I don't know what to do. Can you give me something?"

"Well, what have you been eating lately? Maybe it's time to change your diet."

"Aw, Donny, I don't have time for diets and charts! I've got a script to shoot. Just give me something to make the pain go away, okay? I've got a deadline to meet."

Dr. Belcher sighed. "Sure, Tom. Let me give you a prescription for Zantac. It should help your stomach pain, but if it doesn't, let me know, and we'll step up the dosage, okay? Or we'll switch you to Tagamet. If that doesn't work, though, we'd better run some tests."

"Thanks, Donny. I appreciate it. Anything to get rid of this pain."

"You still taking that Prozac Dr. Mellow prescribed for your stress and depression, Tom?"

"Yeah--just got the prescription refilled on the way over here. I don't know what I'd do without it."

"I'd like to see you learn to do without it. You need to de-stress, my friend--maybe take some time off to relax. You've been working awfully hard lately without a break, and I've been reading some not-so-good news in the *Journal of the American Medical Association* that makes me want to see you get off the stuff real soon. We need to talk about this, okay?"

"Sure, sure--when I get done with this blasted shoot. No, then I go on location. Well, I'll see you sometime later this summer, okay, Donny? Can't let anyone down--I've got a million people depending on me, expecting another hit."

"Right. Well, Tom, I've probably got a waiting room full of some very demanding sick people who need me, too."

"You think I don't know it? I gave up over an hour of my precious time waiting for you out there...and I'm your friend."

Dr. Belcher sighed again. "Lately it seems like everybody either calls in with an emergency and wants a miracle cure, or they come in after eating a pepperoni pizza and want a 45-minute explanation of why they have gas. Some days are so...you just don't know. I get so stressed myself that I have to go pump iron or take a long walk to ease the tension. Oh well, not your problem! Gotta go. Call me and let me know how the prescription works."

Tom DoRight took his Zantac faithfully. For a while it eased his stomach pain and he felt much better--until, that is, he got hit by recurring bouts of the flu, either preceded or followed by a cold. His energy level hit an all-time low, he was always short of breath--he just plain felt lousy. He had his secretary make an appointment to see Miles Tugo, M.D, another good friend. Miles was an internist who could surely be trusted to come up with some kind of pep pill--maybe even an antibiotic to fight off the recurrent flu.

"Miles! Man, am I glad to see you. I'm having all sorts of problems I hope you can fix for me."

"Such as...?"

"Can you give me anything to pep me up? My tail end is dragging like crazy these days."

"Have you considered getting out of your chair and doing a little exercise? It would make you feel better, give you more pep. You ever heard of 'use it or lose it?'"

"Aw, Miles, I don't have any time for pumping iron or plodding along a treadmill. I'm a busy man. Besides, I exercise every day--running all over looking for actors, getting things settled. I hardly feel as if I sit down at all. That's why I'm so tired! I need something to feel better now, not some down-the-road exercise lecture."

"Okay, Tom, I'll write you a prescription for something that should give you more energy immediately--but I'd also like you to get more sleep and take better care of yourself. You still haven't quit smoking, have you?"

"All right, all right, get off my back already! I will one of these days. When I'm ready."

"Do it before it's too late, Tom."

"I appreciate your concern. Hey, Miles, you remember Dr. Winton Lefter?"

"The orthopedic guy? What about him?"

"He moved to Phoenix last month, and I'd like to see somebody about getting something for the constant ache in my joints I've had lately. He used to give me prednisone, but I took it all. This damned flu! I thought it would get rid of the extra pain I was having, but it didn't. Now I'm out, and the pharmacy won't give me another refill without a new prescription. Can you recommend an orthopedist you know and trust?"

"Try Dr. Frank Lee Bonesky. He's good--my sister goes to him. I think that's probably who Winton would have referred you to, anyway. Nice guy. In the meantime, why don't you drop a few pounds to help yourself along? Your extra weight could be causing your back problems--and you know that's just adding to your stress."

"Right, doc, I'll put it on my list."

Dr. Tugo sighed. "Well, take it easy, please, and make an appointment to come back in about six weeks."

So away went Tom DoRight, thinking he was doing right by his body. He knew his specialists were taking good care of him. Of course, he also knew he had just split the seam on his last good pair of pants.

Maybe I should pick up some salad, Tom thought--but then his car phone rang, and he got involved in a heated discussion with a studio "suit." By the time he got home, all he could think about was scarfing down the dinner his cook had left for him--prime rib, scalloped potatoes covered with cheese, and canned green beans. His meal was interrupted twice with crises at the studio, and once with a stupid phone pitch, so he treated himself to the rest of the chocolate cake left over from his birthday party, and washed it down with a large glass of milk. Then he sat back comfortably in his favorite overstuffed chair--cigarette in one hand, cognac in the other--and watched one of his favorite action movies on his big-screen television. Ah, what a life, he thought as he drifted off to sleep. Yes, Tom DoRight certainly had it made. Until he had a heart attack.

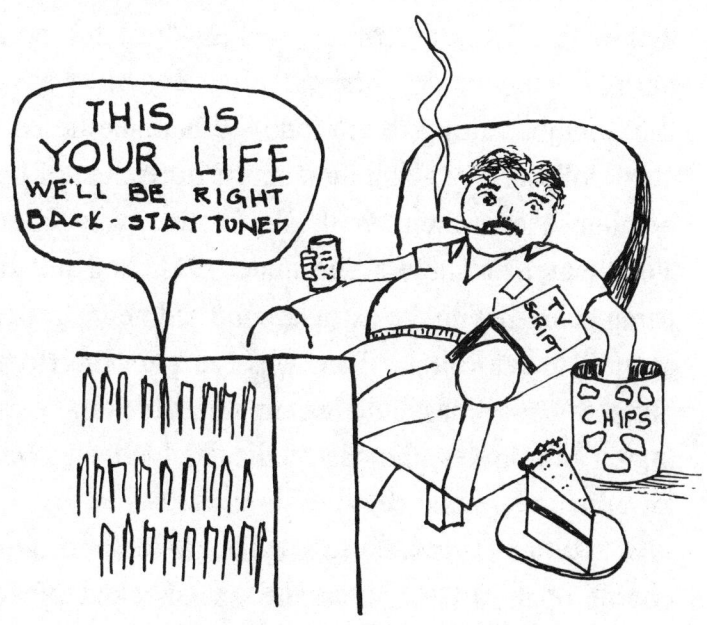

3 - THE CRISIS

Dana was psychic. She knew when the phone was going to ring, and, most of the time, who was on the other end. She knew when to buy and sell her clients' stocks--and she usually turned a good profit. She knew her neighbor Tom pretty well, too, and knew that with all his destructive habits--"just the stuff normal people do," he would say--he was a time-bomb waiting to explode. When she heard a moan followed by a dull thud on the other side of her penthouse apartment wall, she instinctively knew Tom was in trouble. She dialed 911, and let the paramedics in with the extra key she had never gotten around to returning. Tom was lying on the floor, clutching his chest and gasping for breath. In a matter of minutes, the paramedics had whisked him away in an ambulance.

When Dana went to see Tom at the hospital a couple of days later, even she was shocked. Pale, drawn and hooked up to two different monitors with tubes and wires attached all over his body, he looked so unlike the "in control" Tom DoRight she knew and had once loved. He was still too heavily sedated to talk, so she started to leave. She heard talking just outside the room, though, so she lingered quietly behind the door to listen.

"We have to get this 'famous producer' on his feet again quickly," a male voice was saying in a somewhat exasperated tone. "His studio has already called twice trying to get a definite answer as to when he'll be back to work. All those so-called non-invasive treatment methods you're talking about, Mr. Know-It-All-Intern, not only take time before you see results, they haven't even been sufficiently tested, or proven to be legitimate alternatives--especially for patients who have already had an infarction."

"I know he's already had the heart attack, Dr. Strongbeat," a younger voice answered. "It's just that I've been reading some of the things Dr. Bernie Siegel says, and they've really affected me and the way I think I want to practice medicine."

"Bernie Siegel? The name sounds familiar. What's he say?"

"Well..." Dana heard the crinkle of paper. "I wrote this one thing down, because I heard it on TV a couple of months ago, and it struck me like a thunderbolt. He said, 'If you're closed-minded, you can't be scientific, and I'm afraid that's what a lot of so-called scientists are. They think they know the facts, so when you show them something that disturbs them, they say 'beat it' or 'you're absolutely wrong' or 'there's nothing to prove that,' because it confronts their belief system. To me, medicine means the person takes an active part and takes responsibility, has choices, keeps their power--they're part of the team.'"

The older doctor sighed. "Yes, son," he said tiredly, "that is a nice sentiment. Wouldn't it be wonderful if we could get patients to take an active part in their own health care, instead of relying on us to 'fix' their tension headaches, or cut away their poor-habit-induced mistakes. That would be the ideal. And it would be ideal if every doctor had an open mind about everything--of course, then, we'd have a hell of a time practicing medicine, wouldn't we? By the time we sorted through all the options to the point where the patient understood everything, he'd probably be dead. Look, Marxism sounds good on paper, too, but any kind of ideal tends to fly in the face of hard-core, day-to-day reality. The fact is, if we were to go with an unproven treatment with this

I HAVE A CHOICE?!   13

patient, not only would we open ourselves up to getting sued if it didn't work, I can almost guarantee we wouldn't get paid. DoRight's insurance company would never cover anything that hasn't been approved by the AMA, much less its own board of adjusters. Besides, what about patient trust? Patients don't like long-term treatments when they can get fast relief from high-tech surgery." After another sigh, the doctor's tone became crisp once more. "Now, Dr. Cutter, what about this colon problem?"

"Ah, yes, the biopsy came back. Definitely positive. From the scope and other tests, I think we're looking at about nine inches."

"Nine inches involved," the intern asked, "or nine inches that have to come out?"

The oncologist made an impatient noise. "You have a problem with treating cancer, too? Do you want this patient to die?"

"Not at all. I just think there must be other ways to treat his colon problems and heart condition than cutting him open. There are so many risks involved in surgery."

"Oh, Good God!" Dr. Cutter exploded. "Of course there are risks in surgery! How about the risk of not having surgery--highly probable death? Sure, there are other treatments--long-term diet control, stress reduction, life-style changes, even chelation therapy. They're not going to work with a patient like this. How did you get an internship here with all your cockamamie ideas? We don't have time to educate you on the realities of medicine with every single patient. Wake up and look around you, for God's sake! Most patients want immediate relief, immediate healing--and they want it without having to change a blessed thing about the way they think, act, or live. I've seen it time and time again--the guy with terminal lung cancer who's still sneaking cigarettes. The woman with a dozen different stress-induced conditions who thinks the answer to all her life problems is to take a tranquilizer--or divorce her husband. We're not here to fix their lives. Half the time, they resent us even making suggestions. We're only here to heal what's wrong with them--and we'd better do it right the first time, or they'll take us to court, malign our reputations and maybe even accuse us of attempted murder. Now, if you want to talk about risk, swallow that dose. My recommendation is to remove the cancer-ridden tissue surgically, and I'm going to schedule it for as soon as possible following recovery from the bypass! Next patient!"

4 - THE CHOICE

When Dana came back to the hospital the next morning, she found Tom still hooked up to several monitors, and looking very uncomfortable.

"Hey, neighbor," she said gaily. "You look like garbage."

Tom groaned. "I feel worse. I hate this. It's awful here. It takes forever to get a nurse's attention, and I can't move with all this junk all over me. I feel so violated! I can't even go to the bathroom by myself. I hate it! I'm hurting all over, Dana. You gotta help me. I gotta get outta here...but I feel terrible. What's happening to me? Oh Lord, I just saw that tray go by, and the food on it looks worse than I feel! What am I gonna do, Dana?"

"Listen, Tom! Do you want to take control of your life again? Do you really want to feel better? I mean really better? Without the surgery; without any toxic drugs and their nauseating side-effects; without being a victim, or a guinea pig for the latest drug or technique?"

"You mean *I have a choice?!*"

"Yes, you have a choice! Let me tell you..."

"Why should I listen to you?" Tom cut her off. "You're crazy--everyone knows it. You know I love you, Dana--we all do--but you are weird. Everyone knows that." Tom smiled weakly. "By the way, thank you for saving my life--you did save my life, didn't you?"

"Weird! Now I've heard them all! You know, I did make the phone call--which means you have to listen to me."

"Give me a break! Didn't I say 'thank you?'"

"Yeah, you always say 'thank you,' but this time you have to pay back more. You have to listen."

"Don't start, Dana. I've heard the lecture before. Remember? That night on the beach? I know all about your 'physician heal thyself,' stuff. We all know the one about the lawyer who represented himself in court, and had a fool for a client. How can anyone be his own doctor?"

"But you can, with help."

"Hey, I didn't go to medical school, you didn't go to medical school. Spare me your 'listen to your body's intuition'--that's always been one of my favorites. Good grief! Like my body knows what it wants. Hey, I know what my body wants--and it never wants for anything long."

"Obviously...except maybe some live nutrition. I do know what my body needs, because I listen to the signs it gives me. Why do you think I'm almost never sick? You don't have to go to medical school to nourish and respect your body--or not feed it a lot of empty calories that actually starve it. My body is my temple, so I treat it with respect. I feed it both physically and spiritually."

"Oh, please, I feel lousy enough as it is. Empty calories, body temple, own doctor. God, I'm so tired! I've got the best specialists in the area taking care of me. What else do you want?"

"Look, Tom, I still care for you even though we....that's besides the point. I'm not saying there's no use for specialists. It's just that I heard all those precious specialists of yours talking, and I know what they're going to do. I don't think you're going to like it."

"Like what? Heard who? Talking about what? What'd they say? What's going on? Come on, tell me. If I don't know what's happening, I don't have any control."

"Oh, Tom, Tom, Tom. You've got to learn to

control the situations inside you, not just the people around you. Don't you want to know what caused your problems, so you can eliminate them, or at least stop them from getting worse? You're so intelligent and eager to learn new things all the time."

Tom sank back into the bed with a feeble snicker on his face. "Nice try, friend."

"Look, I know a doctor that can help you--and probably without surgery or drugs. Dr. Feelgood can teach you what you need to know to get healthy, and stay healthy."

"Dana, I appreciate you--really, I do. And I'm sorry it didn't work out between us--really. But your head is in a strange place. Normal people just don't think like you."

"Right. Like I'm the one who needs to lose 50 pounds. Like I'm the one who has just been diagnosed with colon cancer because of my bad eating habits. Like I'm the one who just suffered a heart attack. Not!"

"Who's been diagnosed with colon cancer?"

"You haven't heard? They're planning your future as we speak. You've been scheduled for bypass surgery this Thursday. I don't think they'll cut up your colon at the same time, but I suppose it's always one of the 'options' they might give you.

I HAVE A CHOICE?!

Would that make you think you were really in control of the situation? Deciding if you should be cut open twice, or only once? Deciding if you simply want to live with the nausea and hair loss from the chemotherapy, or the exhaustion of the radiation? Sorry, I don't think much of your choices."

"You're sorry? *You're sorry*?! I have cancer! There's got to be some kind of mistake here, Dana. You must have heard wrong, you vicious bitch! What did they really say--that I have spastic colon or something? I don't have cancer. You're a liar! You're just trying to get back at me for smoking near your patio."

"Tom, I heard it all clearly. They want to take out nine inches of your colon. The biopsy was positive. It's cancer. I'm sorry. I thought they already told you."

"Cancer! How could you do this to me? You're giving me a death sentence! Cancer killed my mother--and my best friend--and my ex-wife--and Helen and Louie and Greg. How can you just waltz in here and tell me something like that? Cut me open? They cut my mother open--and she died not six months later. They gave Helen chemo, and she got sick to her stomach for days on end, lost all her hair, and ended up dying less than a year later. And

Greg--remember Greg? Remember the abscess from the incision because he moved around too much, too soon? Remember how the thing smelled, and how they ended up having to cut all sorts of pieces off him, and...oh, God, Dana! You know how I feel about knives and surgery and that kind of thing! I can't even get an ingrown toenail cut out! And they'd have to put me under anesthesia! Anesthesia! My ex-wife never woke up from the anesthesia. She went into a coma, and lay in that bed like a vegetable for almost two years before she died. I can't have surgery! I could die. I could die!! This can't be real. That's it--this is a dream, a scene from some stupid film. I'm gonna wake up, now! NOW!!"

"Look, Tom, it's not a dream, and unless you make another choice, they have you scheduled to go under the knife for both your heart and colon. If you'd rather leave that as a last measure, I know Dr. Feelgood can offer you other choices, other ways where you can heal yourself."

"I'm not a doctor!" Tom almost screamed. "For God's sake, will you get real for one minute in your life! It's not up to me to heal myself--that's all voodoo mumbo-jumbo! Why do you think we have doctors who study all those years? So they can heal the sick--them, not me!"

"Thomas Elvin DoRight," Dana hollered back, "you are where you are right now because of your attitude! You think it's all your doctors' responsibility to make you better, but what about your responsibility in all this?"

Dana stopped yelling when she saw the pain streak across Tom's face.

"Geez, Dana," he panted. "You're making my chest hurt again."

"Oh, Tom," she said, falling into the chair next to the bed with an exasperated air. "*I'm* not making your chest hurt! No one makes your chest hurt except you. Can't you see that? Can't you see how you always try to make it someone else's fault, but it isn't? You never take responsibility anywhere, Tom, except on the set. It's your body--not mine. It's your responsibility to keep it healthy--not the doctors'. They didn't make you have a heart attack or develop cancer. You did it to yourself, and you know it. Please, please--let me introduce you to Dr. Feelgood. What can it hurt to listen to what he has to say?"

"Oh, right, and let some guru run my life? Eat nerdy food and turn into a weirdo, like you? This is what you mean by having a choice? Some choice! The knife or the witch doctor! At least with a real doctor, I have some control!"

"You're willing to let a bunch of other people dictate what's going be done with your body, when you're going to be cut up in the name of science, what drugs you'll have to take to stay alive or suppress the pain that's trying to tell you something--maybe even dictate how long you're going to live--and you call that having control? What are you controlling? How much money they get to make? How much pain and fear you get to experience? Is that the kind of control you want?"

Tom didn't answer Dana. His fearful stare said plenty.

Dana softened. "I read a great book by Dick Quinn called *Left for Dead*. It's his true story--I'll get you a copy of the book to read while you're recuping here."

"If you liked the book, I'm sure I won't, so don't waste your money."

"Lord, Tom, you are a pain in the you-know-what! Dick Quinn had bypass surgery just like they want to give you. It didn't work for him and doctors wanted him to have another bypass at another great expense--not only to his pocketbook, but to his body's ability to maintain a strong immune system. He decided not to listen to his doctors' wishes since they went against his own and, in desperation, he

I HAVE A CHOICE?!

remembered what was probably an angel in the form of a woman in the park who advised him to nourish his heart with some cayenne pepper. He took some cayenne from his spice cabinet and felt more energy than he had in years the very next day! When he realized it must be the cayenne that had seemed to start his heart pumping him some new energy, his research into natural healing with herbs began. His story is really exciting. He was given a new lease on life in 1978--by the way, he was only 42 when he had a heart attack--and is still speaking on programs all over the country and writing new books. Don't argue with me. I'm gonna get you his book and that's that. And you are going to read it, so there."

"All right. I'm tired, Dana. I don't want to argue right now." Tom fumbled with a match, almost igniting a tube leading into his upper arm.

"All right, I'll let you rest. But why don't you doze off with this thought. Control isn't just what's happening on the movie set, Tom. Real control is about what goes in and out of your body, and how much you do or don't abuse it. Like your smoking--here you are, lying in a hospital bed, looking like something out of a bad sci-fi movie--and you're lighting up a cigarette! Don't you think it's time you finally give up smoking? Look, why don't you just talk to Dr. Feelgood? You saw what he did for Jason Summers."

"Jason? He looks so good these days. I thought he was a-goner last Easter when he found out he was HIV-positive. I still think he should gain another ten pounds, though. Hey, I know who your Dr. Feelgood is--I met him at Jason's office once. He seemed like a pretty down-to-earth kind of guy."

"Will you talk to him?"

"I guess so--provided you don't start hassling me about my smoking. I'm in no shape to handle quitting right now!"

"You're in no shape to keep depleting your oxygen supply right now, my friend. Besides, I can't imagine your cardiologist approves of your smoking, does he?"

"Hey, this calls for no-hassles; that's the deal, take it or leave it."

"Okay. You know, if we call Dr. Feelgood right away, he might even do a consultation here in the hospital before you make any further decisions."

"Fine. What's his number? Oh, and while I'm calling, could you be a sweetheart and find me an ashtray?"

5 - WHAT DID I DO?

Dr. Feelgood agreed to come to the hospital and be re-introduced to Tom DoRight. "I loved your last film," he said, shaking Tom's hand. "In fact, I've liked everything I've seen of your work. You obviously take a lot of care with every little detail of the production. It really shows. I always catch nuances in your movies you just don't find in some other films. You must stay on top of everything."

Although not easily flattered, Tom beamed from under his fog of painkillers at Dr. Feelgood's assessment of his work. Something of a perfectionist, Tom took the most pride in the tiny bits and pieces of his movies--things that most people did not pick up, but that "made" the film for him. He lay back in the bed, appreciating this "holistic" doctor's good taste.

"So, doc, Dana tells me you can offer me more choices than the doctors here at the hospital. I mean, I know I can turn my body over to the surgeons, but...well...I've got this thing about knives."

Dr. Feelgood nodded. "I don't like them either. I used to run with a pretty rough crowd in high school. Saw too much damage up close. That's why I went into medicine to begin with--I wanted to heal, not hurt."

"Yeah, well, when I was a seven-year-old kid at camp, this big bully named Clay used to throw knives at trees," Tom went on. "One day he tied me to a tree near the river, and started throwing them at me, always just missing by a fraction of an inch. A counselor finally heard me screaming and came running. He grabbed Clay just as the last knife left his hand. Needless to say, the bastard's aim was off, and he got me right here in the shoulder...see, look at the scar...it really tore into the muscle. I thought it would never stop bleeding. You know, this shoulder still gives me trouble. You know what else? I don't know why I just told you all that. I tell very few people about my phobias. I guess it's the drugs--or maybe I just feel comfortable with you, doc."

"Thanks, Tom. I feel honored. But you're right--with that kind of a phobia, I certainly understand why you'd want to avoid the knife. I know you're feeling rather hazy right now, but let me ask you a few questions. Do you have any idea what happened to make your body start breaking down?"

"Stress, I guess. What else?"

"Oh, I'm sure stress is one factor, but what else?"

"Okay, so I gotta stop smoking. I've been smoking since I was 15. Hey, it's not an easy habit to kick."

"You're telling me! Still, I think your body is at least as important as that fancy Jaguar I've seen you in."

"Huh? My Jag? I'm more important than my Jag!"

"You wouldn't just turn your Jag over to the mechanics and let them fix whatever's wrong, however they want, would you?"

"Are you crazy? You gotta stay on top of those guys every minute! There's no telling what they'd do. Besides, I tune it special, to keep the engine extra clean, and I change the oil every 1,500 miles--not every 2,500 like they tell you. Geez, if I only listened to them, my baby wouldn't be the classic it is today!"

"Well, isn't turning your body over to other people for them to 'fix' the same kind of thing as dropping off your Jag at the shop and walking away?"

"You're confusing me, doc. Geez, it's hard to

think with all these painkillers in me--they fuzz up my mind."

"Maybe you should listen to the pain, Tom, instead of trying to repress it."

"Huh?"

"Pain is your body's way of telling you something is wrong and needs correcting--it's not just an arbitrary inconvenience, or a malicious conspiracy to distract you. You should listen to your body, Tom. It's trying to tell you it needs attention."

"Hey, I pay attention. I went to the doctor. I'm here, aren't I? Lying around when I should be at the studio getting film in the can. I called you--even though Dana cornered me into it, I did call. I'm trying to do the right thing, whatever that is."

"I know you are, Tom, just as I know your doctors are trying to do the right thing for you, despite your efforts to hinder them. They probably felt they had no choice but to give in to your pressure for immediate relief of whatever condition ailed you at the time, didn't they? You didn't pay the kind of attention to the little details of your body and your life that you give to your movie-making. I can't believe you would ever film a scene without having control over every little detail, every minute nuance of the set, the lights, the sound, the camera angle, the actors' delivery--even the kind of sandwiches waiting on the side of the set."

"Of course not--I'm the guy in charge! It's my butt on the line if it doesn't all come down right--and on budget. I hire the best, but I've always got to have the final say."

"Well, it's your butt on the line--really on the line--here, too. What would you do if your sound man told you there was only one way to mike the set, but you weren't happy about it?"

"I'd show him the error of his ways--and if he didn't get it the way I wanted it, I'd do it myself. Hey, I can do every single job on that set!"

"My point, exactly, Tom. Yet, you are willing to turn your body--your personal Jag, your life's film, so to speak--over to someone to do with as they see fit, whether you approve of it or not."

"I never thought of it that way, doc. I'll tell you this--I absolutely hate the thought of surgery. Have you got something in your witch-doctor bag that'll get me out of this?"

Dr. Feelgood laughed. "Yes, I think I do, although every patient is different. For some, especially those whose dread of cancer is so overwhelming they can't cope with the idea of it, I would recommend going ahead with the surgery, and working my program in conjunction. But with your fear of knives...."

"Look, doc, let's be real--I don't fear knives, I'm terrified of them. I'm petrified. I can't even stand the thought of them. I'm...I'm...I'm...."

"Like I said, with your fear of knives, I think you should try to work the program alone, first. Surgery is always an option we can save for a last resort. Actually, you're probably lucky you are so scared of having an operation, Tom. Otherwise, I doubt you would listen to me, even though in your heart, you know I'm making sense. That's okay, though. Sometimes, the best of us have to back into doing the right thing. For now, let's just get you out of the hospital intact."

6 - BACK TO SCHOOL

Tom left the hospital against medical advice and staff protests, and Dana took him to Dr. Feelgood's office. Dr. Feelgood explained that a lot of their time together would center on teaching Tom how to take care of himself. It seemed easy enough.

"Tom, let's start with the basics of what makes the body work."

"Food, water and a lot of love, right?"

"Yes, you need those, too. But what I want to talk about is **energy**. All bodies are energy machines. All living things are energy machines. When everything is running at ease in a body, the energy flows smoothly. If something is not at ease in a living body, the energy is blocked in that area. The blockage causes pain, which generally builds up until the circuit is 'repaired,' and the energy can flow smoothly again. Energy can often be reintroduced to a blocked area by massaging where it hurts, like when we rub a sore muscle, or get a body massage.

I get chiropractic adjustments, or go for acupressure or acupuncture when I don't have time for a full massage. All these techniques release blockages--open up the circuits--and let the energy flow smoothly."

Dr. Feelgood smiled at the look on Tom's face. "Does any of this make sense to you?"

"Yeah, sure, okay, whatever. Listen, doc, don't get too wacko on me, will ya? I mean, it sounds logical, in a weird sort of way, but so what? What does any of that have to do with me? I can't very well massage my blocked arteries, or rub away the cancer in my colon. I thought you were gonna give me a program. Can't you just write it up for me?"

Dr. Feelgood smiled again. "No, of course you can't just reach in and massage the inside of your body. And I know you simply want me to hand you a sheet of paper with a program, and let you go on your way. Unfortunately, that approach wouldn't get you very far. Didn't any of your doctors ever mention your eating habits, cutting down on your workload, or any other lifestyle changes? I'm sure someone must have handed you a diet sheet somewhere along the line."

Tom DoRight moaned. "Hey, I'm a busy man. Who can worry about that kind of thing at work?"

"Well, Tom, that's why I'm not just going to write it up for you--it wouldn't work. That kind of imposed regimen seldom does. People who are busy or in pain have enough on their minds without trying to keep track of something essentially meaningless to them. Besides, if I were to tell you your life depended on only eating and doing what is on one sheet, and avoiding what is on another, how would that make you feel?"

"I'll tell you how it'd make me feel," Tom said, his voice rising with anger. "Like I'm behind bars, that's how. I've tried it. What, you think I've never tried to follow one of my doctors' diets? You think I don't read about all the latest stuff in the papers? I've given it a go before--tried to stay off sugar and coffee and chocolate and beer and all the rest. I felt like a bloody prisoner in my own body. I couldn't eat anything I liked, and I didn't like anything I could eat. If that's where all this is heading, just forget it. I'd rather go under the knife than live like that. It simply doesn't work!"

Dr. Feelgood laughed out loud this time. "Tom, you're wonderful, you really are. You're always making my points for me!"

Tom's anger dissipated as quickly as it had risen. "Huh?"

"What you have described is just what we want to avoid. I don't want you to feel like a prisoner again. Psychologically, the worst thing I could do is try to force you to make changes against your will. Now, I'm not going to pretend that you won't need to make some changes--you already know you will, if you want to get better without surgery. But you will be making your own decisions--educated decisions. My purpose here is to help you learn some basic simple facts about what's going on in your body, why you've developed these problems, and why and how your body reacts to what you eat and do. This way, when you are faced with a choice about what to eat, or what to do, or how to proceed, you can make an educated decision, not simply feel compelled to follow some seemingly arbitrary orders out of panic or fear. You deal with people all the time, don't you, Tom?"

"Hey, it's only my life."

"Exactly. So you know that you can get much better results out of someone who really understands his job, and knows how to make the right decisions every step of the way, than you would out of someone who has only read about the work, and has to be watched every second, right?"

"That's why I hire only the best. I've always

I HAVE A CHOICE?!   35

believed in specialists."

"Okay, then--we're going to make you into a specialist on your own body. You're going to learn what you need to know about making it work correctly and helping it heal itself, so you can make the right decisions every step of the way--and if you don't, you'll know exactly what you're doing that way, too. Now, does this make sense?"

"Okay, doc, you're intriguing me. I know you're just trying to bamboozle me by speaking my own language, but I said I'd give it a shot, so I will. Go ahead--what does 'energy' have to do with my heart disease?"

Dr. Feelgood smiled again. "I guess I'd better make this good, huh? Well, to start with, you are an individual energy machine, with your own personality, and your own individual likes and dislikes, as well as your own strengths and weaknesses--physically and otherwise."

"So?"

"Treating your disease as separate from you, therefore, doesn't really make a lot of sense. If we work with your whole self, your heart disease--almost anyone's heart disease--can be reversed, as long as we get to it in time. Cancer isn't a death sentence, either--and neither is AIDS, for that matter, although we always hear it's absolutely fatal. The unfortunate part is that more often than not, both cancer and AIDS do turn out to be death sentences."

"They have been for most of my friends and family. I guess since it runs in my family there's just a genetic tendency for us to get it. But I don't wanta die right now. I have too much to do, still."

"Yes, it's a shame, but after 35 years of research, the various arms of the medical community have been unable to find a 'cure' for cancer. As things stand now, one out of every three Americans will develop cancer during his or her lifetime--you're already that one in three, Tom--and one out of every five will die from it. I believe--and a great many other people in the healing arts do, too--that the reason has to do with our traditional American approach to a 'cure.' We keep trying to destroy the foreign organism, rather than heal the body. I think that's backwards. I believe if you make the body strong enough, it will heal itself. I've seen it happen countless times. For example, did you know that every single human being carries cancer cells in his or her body at all times?"

"Everyone?"

"That's right. A cancer cell is actually just an abnormal body cell. We all have them. The reason some people 'get' cancer and some do not is because some bodies get more out of balance than others, and create a hospitable environment for those irregular cells to grow and expand. Cutting out the bad cells does not change the environment that allowed them to grow in the first place. I believe that's just one reason why the so-called 'war on cancer' has been so very disappointing. Another problem is the treatments used to 'kill' the cancer--surgery, chemotherapy, radiation. They often leave the body so debilitated and weak, it cannot fight off the slightest infection, or any other malfunction. To my mind, the number of deaths averted by these treatments is too few to justify their widespread use. You and I are going to work on your problems from a completely different angle."

"Hey, I've known people who have been 'cured' by all that stuff you're dismissing."

"Oh, yes, of course. Technology has made great strides. But I would be willing to put money on it that if you talked to those people who have been 'cured,' you'll find that in addition to chemotherapy and radiation, they made some changes in their lives to make their bodies healthier overall."

"Maybe. I have a very lovely friend, Carmen, who was diagnosed with leukemia seven years ago.

She had a few chemotherapy treatments, and was supposed to have a bone-marrow transplant, but her insurance wouldn't pay for it. She got so desperate that she ended up going to some weird doctor who made her become a vegetarian and do a bunch of other strange things. She actually recovered faster, I think, than the other doctors told her it would take from the transplant. I remember, she said she'd gotten back into balance again, and that's what really helped her recovery. Is that the kind of stuff you mean?"

"Are you talking about Carmen Gutlieberz?"

"Yeah, you know her?"

"Yes, I'm that weird doctor she saw seven years ago that suggested she make the lifestyle changes that have her down from a size 16 to a size 8. She stopped by to see me today, as a matter of fact. She had just done 40 laps in the pool."

"She does 40 laps every day! She's amazing. You know what she told me recently? Not one of her five doctors can find a trace of the leukemia. She looks better today than she did 10 years ago--and she says she feels better, too. Unbelievable, when you think about it!"

"Not so unbelievable. The human body and the logic with which it works is a wonderful miracle.

I HAVE A CHOICE?!

Are you aware of the kind of diet Carmen follows?"

"All I know is she's a lot like Dana. She won't mix this with that, she checks every ingredient with the chef when she's at a restaurant, and she eats a lot of rabbit food."

Dr. Feelgood broke into laughter. "Oh, Tom, I think we're gonna get along just fine."

"Well, doc, at least you've got a good sense of humor. I'll see ya next time."

"Where are you going?"

"Isn't our time up?"

"Ah, that's right--you're used to 5-minute check-ups. No, no, I always set aside at least 3 hours for an initial session with a new patient, as long as the patient is strong enough. We need time to go over some basics. You'll be seeing a lot of me for a while. This is really a training program you're going through--you've got quite a lot to learn. At times, I'll have you come in with some of my other patients, so you can get some positive feedback, and find out how they've managed with various things you're having difficulty with. This is no come-back-and-see-me-in-six-weeks program."

"Wow, I really didn't know what I was getting into. Do we at least get to break for lunch?"

"Absolutely. But first, let's get back to

traditional American medicine, and your cause-and-effect expectations."

"My expectations? How do you know what I expect?"

"We all have expectations. We throw the switch (cause), and we expect the light to come on (effect)."

"Yeah..."

"Cause and effect. If the TV doesn't go on, we know the cause probably has to do with a burned-out picture tube. That's a really condensed version of what I think has happened to American medicine. We go to the doctor, and we expect his pills or treatment to make us better. What's more, we expect it to happen on its own--the magic is in the pill or the therapy."

Tom blinked a few times and looked away, but Dr. Feelgood continued. "Now, don't get me wrong when I talk about having little justification for certain treatments offered by Western medicine--obviously, I'm not talking about all treatments. After all, look at the incredible advances American medicine has made in mental illness, life-saving burn treatments, skin grafts, prosthetics, eye surgeries that return vision...the list goes on and on. And where would we be without Western medicine's diagnostic techniques, the most advanced in the world? Laser surgeries, too, as well as fertility treatments, and..."

"I get the picture, doc. I thought you were against regular medical doctors all the way around."

Dr. Feelgood smiled. "Never did I say that. We're all here to work together to make humanity more comfortable. I know I sometimes sound anti-American Medical Association, but actually, I simply disagree with drugs that only suppress symptoms, or with automatically cutting or burning things out that are foreign to the body. When it comes to simple living, doctors are always pressured by their patients to get them back on their feet immediately--patients expect 'instant relief' from whatever is causing their discomfort. Cause and effect. As a result, the 'necessity' for antibiotics, painkilling drugs and surgery has grown way out of control, mostly, I think, because people expect miracles to come in the form of a pill or capsule, and aren't willing to look for the answers the body has to offer."

Dr. Feelgood started pacing and gesturing to an unseen audience. "Look at the facts: since the discovery of AIDS in 1983, few AMA-sanctioned treatments have been found to be effective. Those that do provide some temporary relief have since been proven highly toxic, while still not representing a cure. And, of course, cancer research has been going on a lot longer than that with no miracle cure found. Now, I'm not blaming anyone--because there is no one single anyone to blame. Government agencies constrain research by offering funding only under limiting guidelines, because they have to justify every single cent they pay out, and there is always someone who questions anything not strictly "by-the-book." As a result, though, researchers find themselves under-funded and, subsequently, understaffed, so their work takes years longer than it might, and is then held up to scrutiny by people who don't necessarily have the backgrounds to understand what they're reviewing. The whole system is a mess..." The doctor took a deep breath. "But don't get me started on all this.."

Tom shook his head. "No, that's okay, doc, I'm fascinated. After all, that's why they're trying to change the health-care system now."

"Change the health-care system!" Dr. Feelgood slammed his fist into his palm. "Do you realize what those changes are going to do? I'll tell you one thing they won't do, and that's look to alternative approaches, especially those that utilize non-aggressive strategies."

He stopped and sat down. "Look, Tom, I'm getting off the subject, but I want to make one thing clear. I'm here to look at your entire picture--not just to prescribe drugs that suppress your symptoms, and make your condition worse by ignoring the cause. America doesn't realize it yet, but this is what real health-care reform is all about: marrying the good of traditional AMA medicine with the good of traditional Eastern medicine, as well as homeopathy, acupuncture, herbal therapy, naturopathy, and various other traditions--into one health-oriented, rather than health-treatment philosophy. But that's politics, and I'm getting too far off the track. For now, what you need to realize is that real body healing takes place over an extended time. You did not get sick overnight, and you won't get well overnight, because I won't give in to your pressure to give you a quick fix. You wouldn't want one anyway--that's why you left the surgeries behind, right? So, let's get down to what's actually going on in your body."

7 - THE STATE OF DIS-EASE

Let's start off by talking about **ease** and **dis-ease**. Right now, your body is in a dis-eased state. Simply put, most illnesses are breakdowns of one type or another in the body's immune system. That's true even of AIDS and cancer, although they are more profound breakdowns than the norm. Treatment for any disease, therefore--including AIDS and cancer--has to focus on re-building the immune system through nutrition, exercise, rest and stress control. Sadly, a lot of the drugs that suppress symptoms and/or fight our 'diseases' actually decrease, rather than aid our immune-system efficiency."

"Like the old joke, huh? If the disease doesn't get ya, the cure will."

"Right. Heart conditions, AIDS and cancer are states of non-ease, or non-health. AIDS and cancer, in particular, are anaerobic diseases. "

"Anaerobic--doesn't that mean no oxygen?"

"Right again. AIDS and cancer cannot live in

the presence of pure oxygen. To live, act and occur--to put the body at 'dis-ease'--they need an environment absent of free oxygen. Introducing pure oxygen to a dis-eased body rebuilds its immune system, which, in turn, decreases the extent of the 'friendly' environment for cancer or AIDS. How much the body recovers depends on the amount of re-oxygenation that occurs in each cell."

"So, how did my body get so 'uneasy?'"

"I hate to have to put it this way, my friend, but frankly, you've spent a lifetime abusing your body's natural defenses, and now you're paying for it. For instance, how many fresh, raw fruits and vegetables do you eat each week?"

"Raw? Why raw? I don't like raw food. Who knows what kind of germs you're eating if the food isn't cooked enough?"

"Don't you ever eat salads?"

"Well, yeah, occasionally. And I see from your look that occasionally is not often enough, huh?"

"Afraid not. Many foods lose their oxygen when heated to 120oF. Cooking destroys all their natural enzymes. If a person eats mostly heavily cooked or processed foods, his or her body will eventually become weak and fall into a dis-eased state. It may not be a drastic disease, but, then again, it may. Eating poorly is like shooting craps with your health. The odds are always in the house's favor--and the house, in this case, is disease, not health."

"Oh, great. Isn't there any way to change the dice?"

"Absolutely. One excellent and easy way to counteract your poor eating habits is to exercise. If nothing else, take a daily half-hour walk. Even mild exercise re-introduces oxygen throughout the body. How often do you exercise now? Daily? Weekly? Monthly? Yearly?"

"Hey, I exercise on the set every day--do you have any idea how often I'm chasing down actors and staff who forget when they're supposed to be where?"

"Ah, but do you break a sweat? Do you get winded? Do your muscles feel stretched, and your mind refreshed?"

"Uh...uh, not exactly."

"Then, uh, uh, you're not exactly getting any real, effective exercise. That's one of the first things we'll have to work on. As with everything else, though, before you commit to a program 'just 'cause it's good for you,' you should understand what happens when you exercise, and why things go wrong when you don't."

I HAVE A CHOICE?!   47

"I guess that's why Dana made me bring a notebook. I'm ready--fire away."

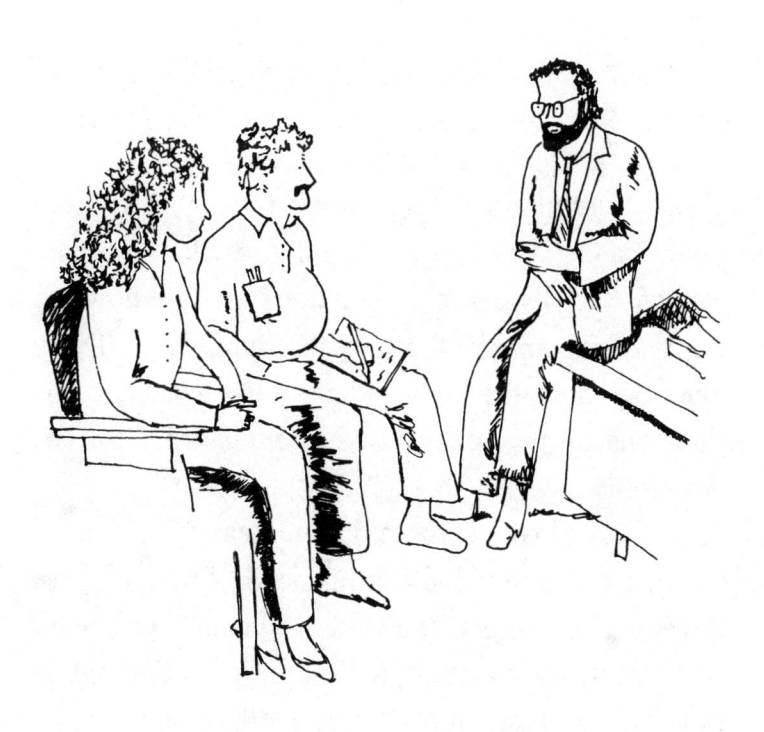

8 - BODY MAINTENANCE

"Let's talk about that Jag you're so proud of."

"A classic, doc, a classic."

"I remember when we first met you told me you'd had it in the shop twice that week. You take care of every little detail. You don't let it go down in any way. **Exercise** is exactly the same thing. Daily exercise gives the body a daily tune-up, and keeps your energy machine in top running order for the duration."

"Until we get too old, you mean."

Dr. Feelgood shook his head. "Actually, we never have to get too old. Haven't you ever wondered why some people look so spry at 90, while others look so old at 57? If you talk to them, you'll probably find the 90-year-olds have reasonably healthy habits, including, just as a matter of course, taking a daily walk. People like Samuel Goldywn, who lived to 90-something, took a walk every day, and had full use of all his faculties for the complete length of his very long life."

"Sam Goldywn? What a powerhouse he was! One of a kind," Tom said with obvious admiration.

"Look around--there are people like that everywhere. You see, part of the marketing strategy for many products is to convince us that as we get older, we naturally get sicker, more infirm, and less alert--regardless of what we do. Our entire society has become convinced that our bodies will eventually age and become decrepit, because God made us that way. But it's just not true! Muscles and bones do not have to age. You can increase or maintain muscle mass as you get older. As a matter of fact, muscle mass declines with age *only if you don't exercise your body*. Look at Jack LaLanne still today. Awesome man, with a very buffed body, and I think he's somewhere in his eighties."

"You know, I heard some guy on a talk show saying this same stuff, just a couple of weeks ago. Some strange name...Deep-end Junkrot?"

"You're thinking of Depak Chopra and his best-selling *Ageless Body, Timeless Mind*," Dr. Feelgood filled in. "An excellent reference book for learning more about the concepts behind what we're talking about. I strongly recommend it. Getting back to exercise, and looking at your fat reserves, or spare tire, as some call it, I'd venture to say you never lift a finger, do you?"

"Thanks a lot!"

"Fact, man. Look in the mirror. And muscles aren't the only body tissues that thrive on exercise, either. Strong bones not only keep you young, they keep you alive. Exercise helps bones stay strong and thick, which helps you avoid osteoporosis, where the bones lose their density, and become weak and porous, often fracturing from the slightest movement. An estimated 100,000 people--60% of them women--break their hips every year for no apparent reason; at least half of them die within 12 months."

Tom made a face. "Why?"

"Lack of exercise. The good news is, bone mass simply will not decrease if it is being exercised. No matter what the person's age, if he or she exercises, those bones will either maintain or increase their mass. It all depends on the type and amount of exercise being performed."

Tom shook his head in confusion. "You know, doc, for the life of me, I can't see how exercise, a muscular activity, affect *bones*."

"That's because you have not started thinking about the body as a whole, instead of a conglomerate of parts," the doctor said. "Exercise maintains the minerals that are necessary for the strength in bones--minerals that would otherwise, indeed, drain away with age. Physical activity can actually even increase bone-mineral content, since, like muscles, bones become bigger and stronger when more stress is placed on them. When bones and muscles don't get exercised or stressed, they become smaller and waste away--not because we're aging, but because we've gotten lazy. We actually stimulate our own so-called aging process by becoming too busy or too sedentary to be as active as we once were. As the years go by, the old adage 'use it or lose it' takes on a more profound meaning."

"Okay, okay, so I need to start exercising. Yuck! I've never liked repetitive movements. Boring! I really don't know if I can force myself to do it. Isn't there any way to get out of it?"

"Sure, you can die," Dr. Feelgood said with a laugh.

"Oh, thanks."

"Or," he went on more seriously, "to put off the inevitable, you can go back to the hospital and have a couple of surgeries first. You tell me. Has not exercising done anything to improve your health? Instead of drinking booze to loosen you up and give you that relaxing 'high' you look for at night, why not take a brisk walk, get those endorphins pumping through your body, and enjoy the natural high?"

"You know, I've heard the word 'endorphins' bantered around a lot, but nobody's ever told me what an endorphin really is."

"Technically, endorphins are a group of brain substances, also known as polypeptides, that bind to opiate receptors in various areas of the brain, and thereby raise the pain threshold.

"But of course," Tom grinned blankly.

Dr. Feelgood laughed again. "For your purposes, just think of endorphins as natural painkillers manufactured by the brain and released into the bloodstream during exercise, bringing on a 'natural high.' Many people who get used to daily exercise come to depend on that natural high--it's what you'd call a healthy addiction--and exercise faithfully as a result. They get to the point where they don't even feel good if they miss a day or two, because they're not experiencing the endorphins.

"Yeah, I know a lot of exercise freaks."

Dr. Feelgood showed his smile once again. "That's right, Tom, fight the logical course to the bitter end. Listen, besides improving, strengthening and increasing your muscle tone and bone mass, exercise can also help you:

- Lose or control your weight
- Lower your blood pressure
- Lower your triglycerides, or harmful blood fat count
- Raise your high-density lipoproteins, or HDL--the "good" kind of cholesterol--level
- Improve your heart output and efficiency
- Improve the oxygen-carrying capacity of your blood
- Lower your blood sugar
- Regulate your insulin responses

"*All* these 'side effects' are conducive to a long and active life. *Inactivity*, on the other hand, lowers your odds for a long, healthy life. It actually doubles your risk of premature death from heart disease. Look at yourself, and the kind of shape you're in right now because you've let your body down."

"I wish you hadn't said that--because I was just thinking that's what I've done. I've let myself get sick--maybe even helped myself get sick. Oh, God, so it's back to the treadmill and weight-room, huh?"

"Not necessarily. Certainly in the shape you're in right now, I would advise moderation. Write that word down--I'll be using it a lot as we go on. Moderation. You don't necessarily have to throw yourself into rigorous exercise to recover and maintain good health. A good brisk walk can do all those things I mentioned before. And there is no excuse for you not to go walking."

"Should I be writing all this down?"

"That's not really necessary, either, because it isn't the actual facts I want you to remember, so much as the idea that you cannot possibly expect to live a long and healthy life if you don't exercise. Something as simple as walking 30 minutes a day, three times a week, will oxygenate your entire body. Because your heart will pump more blood per minute, you will automatically increase the amount of oxygen that reaches all your tissues. It doesn't matter how old you are, or how sedentary the rest of your day is--just that little bit of walking will make a marked difference in your overall health."

"Enough that I don't need surgery?" Tom hedged.

"All by itself, while you still pig out on junk food?" the doctor hedged back. "What do you think?"

"Okay, okay. I just wanted to give it a shot. Nothing ventured, nothing gained, as they say."

"Exactly--again! Nothing ventured physically,

I HAVE A CHOICE?!

exercise-wise, nothing gained--like health, like recovery, like less pain, like long life, like..."

"I get it! So, go on. What else?"

Dr. Feelgood smiled. "In 25 words or less? Let's just leave it with this: age does not destroy our capacity to exercise--**not** exercising does. Most people today feel exhausted and even a little bit under the weather most of the time, because they're stressed out, eating lousy food, and sitting around all day instead of getting out and stretching their bodies. Madison Avenue would love to have us believe the only way to feel better is to buy their myriad of products, but the fact is, exhaustion is often nothing more than the body being out of tune with itself. Where we used to run, climb, carry, lift, crawl and work hard to accomplish the easiest of tasks, we now rely on 'modern conveniences' that help us with--or totally free us from--such labors. Sure, we've simplified our lives, but look at the damage we've done to our bodies!"

"I guess no one has been doing me such a great favor, waiting on me hand and foot, huh? That is...**I** haven't done myself such a great favor, **letting** people wait on me hand and foot. When I get off disability and back to work, I'll be my own gofer!"

"Now I'm hearing something I like!"

"Good. I'm going home to take a walk--then a nap. I'll see you again, when?"

"Tomorrow."

"Tomorrow, then."

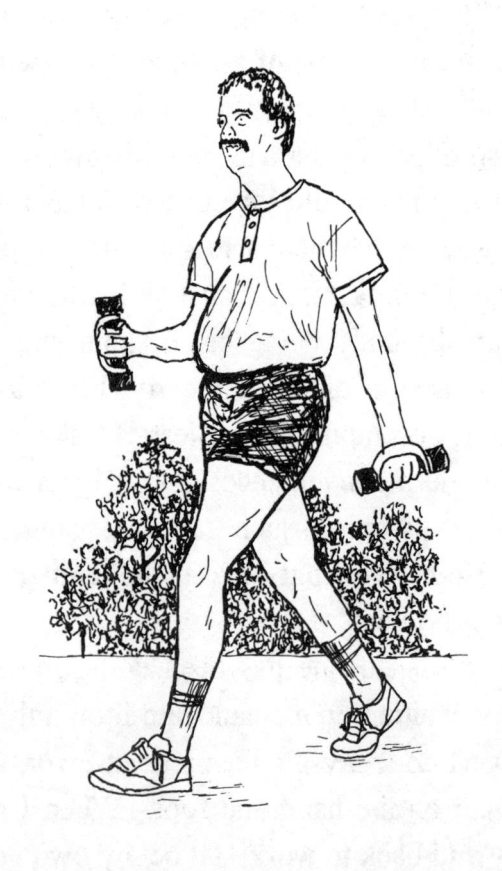

9 - VITAL ENERGY

Tom DoRight showed up at Dr. Feelgood's office for his next appointment looking tired and grumpy. "How are you feeling today, Tom?"

"Lousy. I walked 30 minutes, like you told me. I could barely breathe by the time I was done, practically had to crawl to my apartment, and crashed for the rest of the day. I didn't wake up until a couple of hours ago. This is supposed to be good for me? Remember, I've got a heart problem!"

"Yes, and you've exercised your heart--worked that muscle, which is what the heart basically is--for the first time in Lord-only-knows-how-long. Don't worry, what you did was good for you. And I'd like you to do it again this evening. But first, let's get to our lesson for the day."

"Wait, before you get into all that, can we talk again about cooking foods? You said you destroy the nutrition in food whenever you cook it, right? You've got me afraid to eat. Now that can't be right."

"No, this time, you're not quite on the money. I said that cooking many foods above 120o Fahrenheit destroys the **enzymes** in it. Perhaps I should have said that **the way** many foods are cooked destroys the nutritional integrity of the foods. Actually, food is the topic of the day, so we might as well start there as anywhere."

Tom pulled out his notebook. "Okay, I'm ready."

"Here's how it works. **Enzymes** are the **life** in food--they're what keep the human body healthy. Our bodies are made up of billions of microscopic cells, whose very existence depend on live enzymes to digest the food we eat, and absorb the food's nutrients into the blood."

"So if I cook any of my food, I'm...I can't...my body won't.... I don't get it."

"Wait, let me get it all out. Enzymes are actually the life of every living thing. They're what cause seeds to sprout into plants, and cause plants to grow and bear fruit or flowers. Without enzymes, no plant, animal or human could live. Enzymes are intimately involved in the action and activity of every atom in every form of life. Where there is life, there are enzymes. Since the intangible of 'life' itself cannot be explained, it is often referred to as the 'vital force' or 'cosmic energy.' Enzymes, therefore, are also known as the vital force or cosmic energy in the body--without them our bodies will simply die."

"So, what do you want me to live on?" Tom demanded with a hint of panic in his voice. "Carrot sticks and celery stalks? I know my life is at stake, but let's be real--I'll never pull it off."

"Hey, slow down, boy," Dr. Feelgood soothed. "Remember that word, moderation? I'm not asking you to give up all cooked foods. I'm letting you know it's time to start thinking about adding some raw, uncooked foods to your daily diet. **Adding**, not necessarily **replacing**. At least not at this point."

Tom's sigh of relief shook the room. "Adding. Adding." His face seemed to clear a bit. "Okay, that I can live with."

"That's the whole idea."

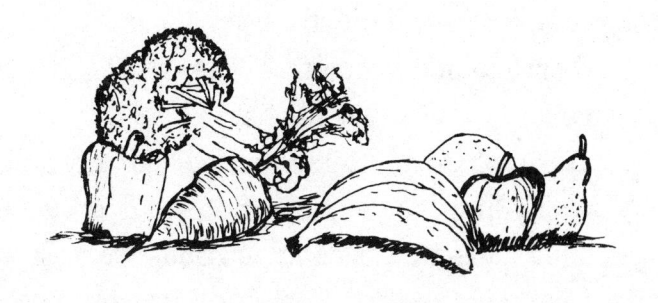

10 - LIFESTYLE ADJUSTMENTS

After Tom drank a glass of water and calmed down, Dr. Feelgood started again. "Let's talk a little about your lifestyle, Tom. Tell me again how old you are."

"Just turned 45."

The doctor grinned. "A great age. Too old to fool around any more, but still young enough to spring back and recover your body's strength."

"And not have to live on carrot sticks."

"And not have to live on carrot sticks. But--and here comes the stuff you've been dreading--you are going to have to get rid of some stuff you're used to if you want to get your strength back, and overcome these dis-eases."

Tom readied himself. "Yeah, go ahead," he said guardedly. "Give me the list."

"Okay, here goes: refined foods of any kind, such as anything containing white flour or white sugar, and cigarettes, alcohol, caffeine, excessive dietary fat such as what you find in many meats, cheeses and butter. And it's always wise to avoid pre-packaged foods packed with preservatives. Also avoid exhaustion."

"Yeah, yeah, go on..."

"For now, that's it."

Tom's mouth dropped open. "That's it?"

"For now. One step at a time, remember? These habits wreak havoc in a healthy body--you know what they've done to your body. Well, they're doing it to a lot of bodies. Look at life these days. Forty years ago, we didn't have burger stands on every other corner in every city and town. Foods weren't as 'fast' or processed as they are now--and people weren't able to consume so many non-nutritional substances on such a regular, daily basis as they can today. What has our do-it-fast, eat-it-fast society done for us? A lot of debilitating, once-rare dis-eases--like your heart disease, or arthritis, multiple sclerosis, cancer, even AIDS--have now become common, everyday occurrences. It's only in recent years, for example, that doctors have made the connection between fast, processed foods and the incredible leap in the number of people who suffer from asthma and allergies."

"How do asthma and allergies relate to all of this?"

"Allergies are just one result of immune-system breakdown. An allergy occurs when the body loses its ability to tolerate certain items it comes into contact with. Asthma can often be attributed to the same cause."

"You mean food used to be healthier?"

"Significantly healthier. It wasn't all sprayed with pesticides or fungicides to protect it from bugs and fungi, or overcooked, processed, chemically preserved to increase shelf life, hormonally enhanced...."

"Why don't they teach us this stuff in school?"

"They did teach you about diet in school, remember?"

"I remember something...I don't know--something about the four basic food groups."

"Right. Which doesn't have as much to do with education as it does with advertising."

"Advertising? In grade school?"

"Let's look at dairy foods, for example. Most of us learned from early childhood that dairy products are one of the necessary four basic food groups--'a lesson in good food for good health' that has been promoted by the dairy industry for years."

"'Drink four glasses of milk every day, or no dessert,' my mom used to tell me."

"Yeah, mine, too. Unfortunately, the idea that four daily glasses of milk were good for us wasn't education, but advertising. In reality, cows' milk is the most mucus-forming food we could possibly consume. Even the AMA admits that drinking milk encourages and aggravates colds, runny noses, asthma, and tonsil, adenoid and bronchial troubles in both children and adults."

"Yech. Mucus. I'm always full of it. I blow my nose constantly--but I almost never drink milk. Well, unless I have chocolate cake. I mean, you gotta have milk with chocolate cake, right?"

"Do you eat ice cream?"

"Occasionally."

"Use cream in your coffee?"

"Well, yeah."

"Put sour cream on your baked potato? Use milk on your cereal? Cover your salad with a creamy dressing, like blue-cheese, or ranch, or creamy Italian? Eat cheeseburgers?"

"Message received. So how do I get rid of all this mucus? Exercise? Maybe put in an extra 10 minutes a day?"

Dr. Feelgood laughed. "Wouldn't that be great? No, I'm afraid it doesn't work quite that way. You might consider drinking fresh carrot juice, though. Fresh, I repeat, not the canned stuff. You can either get a juicer and make it, or buy it at the store. Your local natural-foods store will always carry it, and a number of supermarkets are starting to carry it on a regular basis. Check the date carefully. You only want to drink juice that is less than three days old. After that, it leaves an icky taste in your mouth."

"Carrot juice?"

"Yup. Carrot juice is one of the greatest aids for eliminating mucus. It flushes the gunk out of all your cells, not just your nasal cavities. Mucus builds up everywhere. In fact, when you clean out your cells with carrot juice, it often helps you take off weight. Not that the gunk weighs a lot, but it's sticky..."

"Yech!"

"...and so it holds the extra fatty material in the cells."

"That's gross!"

"I guess it is. See, cows' milk is made for calves to drink; they have the digestive systems to tolerate their mothers' milk. Humans don't. It's that simple."

"Did the milk products give me cancer?"

"No one thing 'gave' you cancer, Tom. But

dairy products do help set up that disease-friendly environment we talked about."

Tom shuddered. "Why haven't I read more about this kind of stuff in the papers?"

"Well, it's out there, you just have to be listening. And you will hear more and more about it, because more and more people are finding their way to holistic doctors after they've run through everything the drugstore and pharmacy have to offer for asthma and some other very common allergies. Also, word of mouth travels. If you tell anyone what you're doing with me, some may think you're crazy; others will come out of the woodwork to share their stories with you--don't be surprised by that. We've all been brainwashed from an early age to believe milk makes a body strong. It does have a lot of good nutrients in it. Unfortunately, they're just not in a form we can readily digest. The *Journal of the American Medical Association* has only recently reported on studies that show milk can cause allergies and asthma. It's really not anybody's fault in particular--dairy companies honestly believe their products are 'good for you.' They're simply continuing the pattern they were taught, and passing on what they know to others. As a matter of fact, did you see the special on T.V. produced by John

Robbins? He grew up with the belief that ice cream was healthy for humans, being the son of an ice cream mogul. The special was the same name as the book--'*Diet for a Small Planet.*' And he now promotes a vegetarian diet for health--no meat--no dairy products."

"Well, I'm sick of always feeling sick. And I think you've just explained why, right after I eat dairy products, I often feel like I have a cold--my nose starts running, my throat itches and I start coughing up gunk. The problem is, I lied--I eat a lot of ice cream. I love ice cream. There it is again--my personal loves going against my physical needs. Have you got something in your magic book for this one?"

"Absolutely, never fear. Check out your local health-food or natural-foods store. They've got non-allergy-producing substitutes for a lot of your favorite foods that taste as good, but are made of healthier ingredients. Ice cream and milk are two of the easiest to replace. Look for some of the products made of soy, nuts or rice. If you really crave a tall glass of milk, you can find a variety of substitutions that cause no allergic reactions, have no dairy fats, and are delicious. Plain soy milk, for example, tastes very similar to low-fat milk. You can also find a variety of flavors, such as vanilla or carob, a chocolate alternative, or try nut milks, such as Amazake, almond milk, or rice milks. They're all very nutritious and not at all mucus-causing."

"Yeah, but what if I don't want to go to a health-food store?"

"Check your regular supermarket. More and more of them are carrying alternate products these days. If you can't find Rice Dream in the ice-cream freezer, or soy milk next to the dairy milk, talk to the manager. That's how products get picked up, you know--consumer demand."

"Rice Dream--I've seen that at Jonny's Market. Is it any good?"

"I like it. Try it and see what you think. It's creamy, smooth and cold, just like dairy ice cream, but it isn't as filling or as heavy, and it won't produce mucus in your body."

"Thanks. You know, this is getting more interesting all the time. I'm starting to see what Dana meant when she said I've been limiting my choices. There's a lot more to choose from than I ever could have imagined!"

11 - PREMIUM FUEL

"Let's go on with some more diet basics," Dr. Feelgood said. "I can't say enough about diet. It's far more important than most people realize, even with all the current emphasis on healthy eating. Most of us in the United States are still eating way too much processed food, which is devoid of anything beneficial for our bodies. Even a healthy, exercised body will eventually break down if it's fed a heavy diet of processed foods. Put cheap gas in your car, and just see how long it runs without problems."

"I wouldn't do that to my Jag!"

"Well, Tom, our bodies are much the same--if they're not fed nourishing foods, sooner or later--probably sooner, as in your case--they'll clunk out."

"So is this where you give me the real eat/don't eat list? I knew it was coming sooner or later, I just knew it."

"Now, come on, Tom, it isn't all that bad. You

I HAVE A CHOICE?!

just have to use some common sense--and learn a few things that will give you a bit more sense of what you're doing. For example, to fortify your immune system, you need to cut way down on your fat, and eat more whole foods that are rich in vitamins A, C, and E and trace minerals. Certainly you have to cut out the stuff that is specifically harmful. And this brings us to another of the heavily advertised '4 basic food groups'--**meat**."

"Oh, Lord, here it comes. No more steak, no more hamburgers, no more chops, no more stew, no more hoagies..."

"Absolutely no more hoagies--that is, if you are trying to choose foods that will help you recover and live a long life."

"Oh, right, it's my choice. Well, I guess it is--as much as it's always been. I've just never really understood what the choices meant before. And I'm not going to pretend I understand this one, either. I always thought people needed protein to live, and the best way to get it was through meat."

"Well, yes and no. While you were still growing as a child, you needed much more protein than you do now, as an adult. People have a grave misconception about how much protein adults need, and--although I occasionally run across the exception, such as certain multiple sclerosis patients--meat is not necessarily the only, or even best way to get it. You see, meat is not just the plastic-covered package you pick out of the refrigerated section of the grocery store. Most supermarket meat--notice I say *most*--is from animals who have been grown in factories under horrendous conditions, rather than raised in the field, like we're used to seeing in the movies. Because of production demands, the animals are kept in crowded stalls, unable to move or exercise. They have to get daily hormone shots so they'll grow, and grow quickly. A farm-grown chicken, for example, takes six months to achieve full growth, while a factory-grown chicken only takes six weeks! The chickens are stuffed one on top of another, which results in the factories becoming highly unsanitary, so a lot of them become diseased. Since cows, calves and pigs, for example, are crowded so closely together in similar unsanitary conditions, they also easily become diseased. To keep these chickens and cows and calves and pigs alive until they can reach slaughter, they're sprayed every day with an antibiotic mist, and fed antibiotics in their food. And any cancerous growths found in the carcass are cut out before the meat is neatly packaged and made pretty for the consumer's buying pleasure."

"Blech. I don't think I'll ever be able to chew another hamburger or steak without visualizing your lovely words. Gee thanks!"

"Then chew on this. When diseased meat enters a human body--your body--it compromises the immune system. So many people look to their doctors to make them feel better, when, in fact, all they really need to do is clean up--literally--their eating habits, and stop ingesting what practically amounts to poison. The problem is, medical doctors are not trained to deal with the intricacies of diet therapy. They're lucky if they receive two to four hours of nutrition in medical school. Generally, outside of avoiding spicy foods with an ulcer, or fatty foods with a heart condition, diet isn't even a consideration, much less a major one. Yet ingesting toxic meats that break down the immune system could easily be the cause of many dis-ease symptoms."

"Could that be part of my problem?"

Dr. Feelgood nodded. "Very well could be. We've seen that in less affluent countries than the United States, where meat is **not** a typical food in the daily diet, cancer occurs much less frequently. People who live on what we in America would consider a poor diet--grains, legumes such as beans and peas, and local seasonal vegetables--actually have better cardiac, digestive and overall health than we do in this country. You only find incurable diseases running amok in wealthy countries where the population eats a lot of 'dead foods'. Most times, the answer to what ails us lies in something as simple as diet. Remember, 'we are what we eat.'"

"Doc, I gotta admit...it all makes perfect sense to me as I sit here in your office, but I'm a meat-and-potatoes kind of guy. Please, please tell me I don't have to give up all red meat forever."

"Didn't you just finish telling me you'd have trouble eating another hamburger or steak?"

"Well, yeah, until I can forget what you told me about the factories and cutting out cancerous growths from the meat and then packaging it just like there's nothing wrong with the meat and...anyway, if I'm able to get past thinking about that stuff, will I really have to give up meat forever? I really do like the taste of it."

"Actually, you don't have to give it up forever."

"No lie?"

"No lie. For right now, however, I would suggest you **choose** to refrain from eating it until your system has had a chance to clean out and build up. Later, down the road--remember that word, moderation? If you still choose to eat beef and lamb, buy meat with no hormones or additives, from range-fed cattle or other animals grown on special hormone-free, antibiotic-free farms. You might have noticed you aren't seeing James Garner promoting 'beef as good food' on any more TV commercials."

"Yeah, well, even I know about the quadruple bypass, and his new 'lifestyle.' I guess that kind of quashed things with the Beef Council, huh?"

"He realized meat could never be a part of his diet anymore if he wanted to live. Now his diet consists strictly of grains (lots of pasta) and fresh vegetables. No animal products anymore because they clogged up his arteries too badly. Simple as that. He chose life over beef."

12 - MIX & MATCH

"So, doc, what do I eat?"

"So, Tom, what do you eat now?"

"Well, I have my first cup of coffee and a bowl of cereal with milk and sugar...uh oh, there goes that milk again...and a couple of eggs, 4 slices of bacon, some toast, orange juice...gotta get my daily dose of vitamin C...oh, and an apple, of course. How come my 'apple a day' didn't keep the doctor away?"

"To begin with, do you eat those items in the order you mentioned?"

"Yea, pretty much so. Why? Does it matter?"

"Everything matters. Sugar at any time is bad for a healthy body, much less a weakened body such as yours. It throws the body's blood chemistry completely out of balance. Also, you're putting incompatible enzymes together when you eat all those foods at one time, which causes all of it to sit in your intestines for hours, if not days, longer than it should be there. Your body cannot properly digest or assimilate any of that mixed together--so, essentially, you're not getting any of the nutrition out of any of the food. And, of course, we've already talked about what the milk is doing to your system. I don't want to get started on food combining right now, though--that's a complete session all by itself. In the meantime, I want to know more about what you eat during a typical day."

"Well, okay, when I get to the studio, somebody's usually brought in some donuts, and I have another cup of coffee. My favorites are the glazed and, of course, chocolate. Gotta have my chocolate fix. Lunch-time we have pizza brought in, or I'll have a ham-and-cheese sandwich. Usually something quick--our shooting schedule is really tight. Oh yeah, once a week they have one of those 6-foot-long sandwiches brought in for us to share--cheese, pastrami, turkey, roast beef, salami, pickles, lettuce, tomato, onion, olives--man, they're so good, I'd love one right now...."

Tom caught himself and shot a glance at the doctor's face, but Dr. Feelgood just smiled and nodded.

"Okay, then," Tom went on, "dinner depends on whether I eat in or out. Sometimes I just nuke one of those microwave dinners if I'm home alone. Couple of times a week, my housekeeper will make something and leave it for me--usually a casserole or roast, chops, potatoes...that kind of thing. If I'm out, I'm a sucker for shrimp or lobster--don't know which I like more. I usually have dessert--what am I saying--I always have dessert. Usually something like ice cream, or a little cheesecake, and a touch of cognac, and I see by your expression I'm killing myself, right?"

"Well, yeah, so far. Of course, you already know that, what with your heart condition and the cancer. By the way, the hospital got your release, and sent over your medical records. The cancer is still in the early stage, which is very good news. In other words, now is the time to treat it, before it really gets a grip, and spreads further. You've come to me at just the right time. I've also talked to your cardiologist, as well as your oncologist. I promised both of them you'd stay in touch. They want to monitor your progress. They care more that you heal than how you heal, although I assume they would have preferred you follow their methods of treatment."

"You mean, I have to be seeing all of you guys at the same time?"

"That's right--remember, I talked about **adding**, not necessarily **replacing**? I don't do biopsies, and I don't do treadmill tests. Now, let's get back to your diet, and getting you as excited about energy-giving foods as you are about energy-depleting foods. You were almost drooling when you talked about that seafood, which raises the triglyceride level (harmful blood fat count) in your body."

"I have a friend with M.S. She says she's supposed to eat shrimp or some other seafood every week."

"You don't have M.S. You have cancer and heart disease. Every person's diet has to be tailored to that body's needs. Today's topic is about some foods that will nourish your body, Tom DoRight, rather than just fill you with dead weight. You were right about one thing--you need to change the way you think about food if you want to improve your health and avoid the big knife. You put on your fat--the weight you need to lose--with your very own hands. You've applied the old hand-to-mouth routine far too often, with the wrong foods. Nobody has a natural tendency to carry 50 extra pounds--and it's not God's fault, either. You've been your own worst enemy all your life, my friend. It's time you become your own best friend."

Tom's sigh did not shake the room this time; it

was a sigh of acceptance, not resignation or relief.

"Let's talk about **organic** vs. **inorganic**," Dr. Feelgood said.

"Like 'organic grocery' organic, like I've gotta buy only organically grown foods that have no pesticides on them?"

"That's not a bad idea, but it's not exactly what I meant. Organic doesn't merely refer to food grown without pesticides or fungicides, although that's what's meant when people talk about growing vegetables. But we are also organic--our human bodies are organic, because we have organization to our corporeal masses. So do animals and plants. All our cells are organized into specific patterns that keep us alive. The cells have their own intelligence, and can recognize and assimilate organic matter as it is taken in. Cooking, processing, canning, or pasteurizing, as we've talked about, destroys the enzymes in many foods and juices, converting the atoms of those foods into inorganic, or dead atoms. Dead atoms are hard for our organic bodies to recognize and assimilate. When the body cannot assimilate all the food constantly being shoved into it, it often develops problems as a result. Your colon cancer, for example, is the result of undigested, unassimilated food remaining in the colon, putrefying

I HAVE A CHOICE?!

and rotting where it...."

"Wait," Tom cut in. "In other words, what you're saying is that most of what I eat--even my low-cal microwave dinners with two vegetables instead of one--is actually destroying my digestive system because it has no live enzymes?"

Dr. Feelgood's voice changed. "That's right, Tom. That's what happened."

Tom stared at the floor for a while, and the doctor remained silent. When Tom looked up again, there was a new glass of water waiting on the table next to him.

"Have something to drink, Tom."

Tom did not seem to hear him. "You do realize this is mind-blowing, don't you? I mean, you really have to change everything about the way you look at foods--completely, all across the board."

"Without a good educational foundation in nutrition, which none of us received in school, and a lot of support, nobody can simply change their eating habits. Don't beat yourself up over what you've done--just open yourself up to what you can do, starting right now."

Tom smiled a little, to stop the tears he felt welling up. "Thanks, doc," he said quietly. "You're right, of course. It's just that, all of a sudden, I feel so totally overwhelmed with guilt. Look what I've done to myself! I almost killed myself! And I didn't even know it--I swear to you, I didn't know I was doing it."

"I know that, Tom. And I don't want you going around blaming yourself--that won't get you anywhere. You didn't mean any harm to yourself, heaven knows! You cannot take the blame for not doing what you did not know you should, or for doing what you thought was right at the time. Why don't we take a little break for a while? Go take a walk--the neighborhood around here is safe. The exercise will kick some of those endorphins into your bloodstream, the solitude will let your mind breathe, and you'll feel better. Be back in about half an hour, okay?"

"Okay. I'll be back."

13 - PROPER FOOD COMBINING

Tom came back to Dr. Feelgood's office looking a little better than when he had left.

"Did you have a good walk?" the doctor asked.

"Yeah, I guess. I thought a lot about what you said. All of it. I'll keep up with my cardiologist, and my oncologist and you. And I think I'm going to read a couple of those books Dana keeps pushing at me--about attitude and changing the way you look at things. You're making me realize that a lot of what she's told me through the years is true. She's not so much a nut as I thought. I guess I've been nuts."

The doctor reached out and put his hand on Tom's arm. "I could give you all sorts of platitudes about new beginnings, and how we learn best from our mistakes, but they won't mean anything to you right now. I know this is a painful process--I'm not going to pretend it won't take a while to come to terms with what has happened, and what you have to do to get well. As with anything in life, you can't skip this phase. As you go through it, though, try to remember this: I don't blame you, and I don't think you should blame yourself. Blame is not the point here, and if you dwell on it too long, it could become destructive. Not that you can erase the thoughts overnight--nobody can. But you're still a good person, a fine director, and, from what I've seen, a smart man. You'll get through this--and I'll be there to help you all the way, okay?"

Tom smiled again, this time for real. "Okay, doc. Thanks." He took a deep breath. "Now, you mentioned something about not eating certain foods together. Could we get to that now? I gotta know what I *can* eat."

"Okay, let's start with the basic reasons why food combining is important. To begin with, anything that's not a vegetable or a fruit is considered a **concentrated food**. The problem is, our digestive systems are constructed to handle only one concentrated food at a time. The best thing you can do for your system, therefore, is not eat more than one concentrated food at a time--especially now, while you're in recovery."

"But how can you eat cereal without milk? Oh, that's right, I shouldn't be having milk. Or is there something wrong with cereal, too?"

"Grains are, again, a whole other subject. The point is, eating grains and milk together depletes your body of energy, even though this combination has been advertised as 'the way to start your day' for decades."

"Why does eating them together deplete my energy?"

"Let's take another favorite all-American combination--meat and potatoes--as an example. Two concentrated foods. When the meat, a concentrated protein, hits the stomach, it needs acidic digestive juices to break it down, digest it and assimilate it. When you eat the potato right on top of it...."

"Wait a minute, Doc. The potato is a vegetable, isn't it? So wouldn't that make it a non-concentrated food?"

"Ah, you are listening! Good. But the potato only remains non-concentrated if you eat it raw, so it can retain its high-water content. I wouldn't suggest you go eating raw potatoes, though. They can be juiced in small amounts for their good benefits, but your system is too weak to eat raw potatoes right now. However, if you bake the potato, fry it, sauté it or boil it, it becomes a concentrated starch, because most of the water has been removed. Unfortunately, the digestive juices required to break down the concentrated starch (the potato) are alkaline, not acidic."

"Acid and alkaline. Doesn't sound good. What happens?"

"For a while, not much. Acids and alkalines neutralize each other, so when they meet in the stomach, the digestive process temporarily stops altogether. Then the work begins again, because your body really wants to digest these foods. It musters all its energy to go at them again, manufacturing more digestive juices, which, again, neutralize each other. You might have noticed how, after a large meal, you tend to get rather sleepy. If you've eaten the wrong foods at the same time, your energy is totally depleted by your body's attempt to digest foods that cannot be digested together. This is actually the complete opposite of what food should do--fuel your body so that you become energized. That only happens if you combine your foods properly."

Tom leaned forward, writing hurriedly in his notebook. "Good combinations fuel, bad combinations deplete. Got it." Tom wrote for a while longer. Okay, so if you eat a bad combination, such as meat and potatoes, when do all these digestive juices stop neutralizing each other?"

"The process continues indefinitely--

unfortunately, sometimes until you get indigestion or heartburn. Peristaltic action will eventually move the undigested food out of the stomach and into the intestines, but in the meantime, most of the protein (the meat) putrefies, and the carbohydrate (the potato) ferments, creating toxic acids in your system. You've experienced this--the lay term is bloating, or gas."

"Oh, yeah, I've had that often!"

"Most people run to their medicine cabinets at this point for their heartburn medication, or for some kind of over-the-counter relief from acid indigestion."

"Which wouldn't have been necessary if they'd just combined right, right?"

"Right."

Dr. Feelgood waited a few moments, while Tom scribbled furiously. Finally, he looked up. "I remember Dana once telling me about some friend of hers who had liver damage. She blamed it on improper food combining. I think I told her somebody had combined her wrong."

Dr. Feelgood grinned. "Anyway," Tom went on, grinning back, "she said he had fermented his intestinal tract the same as if he had been drinking alcohol for years. Is that really possible?"

"Very sad, but very possible. Eating more

than one concentrated food at a time causes the food to rot in your stomach, and rotten food can't be digested or assimilated--it just passes through, or gets stored in the cells along the way, which breaks down the intestine's capacity to function even more."

"Yuck. Double yuck. It just seems so hard to eat that way. My mother always made sure every meal--at least every dinner--had some kind of protein, vegetable and starch. She'd make us sit at the table for hours if we didn't finish our potatoes or rice or noodles."

"Well, like all of us, she was doing what she thought best. There's no going back to correct history's wrongs, which is all that is. It's time to learn, instead, to eat only one concentrated food at a time. If you want a potato, or some noodles, or bread, or some brown rice, eat them with a high-water-content food, such as a salad, or steamed broccoli."

"But if you cook the broccoli," Tom read from his notes, "that makes it into a concentrated food."

"Broccoli is a high-water content vegetable, and doesn't convert to starch when heated, like a potato. But it's still best to steam or lightly stir-fry it, because then it won't be exposed to heat long enough to get up to 120oF. You can eat cooked vegetables with concentrated foods, provided they haven't been cooked to the point where they lose their high-water content."

"I'm confused."

"I don't blame you. It can be very confusing at first."

"Will I ever learn it all?"

"With ease, over time. Just don't combine any concentrated food with fruit. Fruit is a high-water-content food, but it can only be eaten by itself. In fact, a good way to start your day is to eat fruit. But you have to be careful, because there are some rules that apply."

"Such as?"

"Eat fruit in the morning before you eat any other foods. Fruits are the cleansers of the body. When you eat them by themselves, first thing when you get up each day, they have the chance to do their cleansing work, which gets rid of the toxins you've stored up in your body. Wait at least half an hour before you eat anything else after you've had any kind of fruit--an hour would be better. Also, _never_ eat melons with any other kind of fruit. As the saying goes, 'eat melons alone or leave melons alone.' Oh, and only eat citrus fruits with other citrus fruits."

"Melons with melons, citrus with citrus. Got

it. Hey, that doesn't seem so hard to remember."

"Nothing is, when it makes sense. By the way, the same goes for proteins. If you want to eat meat--when you're ready, which, I repeat once again, is not now--the only other food group that will combine well with flesh is a high-water-content food. Again, we're talking about vegetables, not starches, that are high in water content, and certainly not fruits. This combination should be compatibly digestible."

"Maybe I should just get my own personal chef like Oprah has--you know, Rosie Daley. Oprah is looking mighty fine lately, isn't she?"

"That she is. And if you can have someone do your cooking that knows proper food combining--especially the type necessary to heal the body from dis-ease, not just lose weight, that might be the way for you to go. I know there are times, Tom, when proper food combining is difficult. You may slip if you have no control over the foods being prepared, such as when you are a dinner guest at someone's home, or in a restaurant that doesn't provide what you request, but you can always ask. Just do your best to eat the right combinations as much as possible to make your healing faster."

"Does that mean if I eat these combinations I'll feel more energy and less gassy?"

I HAVE A CHOICE?!

"Not only will you feel more energy, you'll automatically drop unwanted pounds. When your food is easier to digest, your body has more energy to use elsewhere. Pounds shed when energy is used properly. What we're looking for is to have your body function harmonically, eliminating wastes with ease rather than holding them in a constipated state because foods were indiscriminately thrown into your stomach all at once."

Tom stared at his notes. "Listen, doc, I'm outta here. I've got enough to think about for one night. I'm going home and eat a humungous salad, drink a quart of carrot juice, and do 5,000 jumping jacks. If I'm still alive in the morning, I'll be back."

"Don't forget, I won't see you tomorrow morning. I'll see you tomorrow evening, when you'll meet some of my other patients. So stay alive--they might be able to answer some of your questions."

"I'll come with a list."

As Tom left the office, he could hear Dr. Feelgood chuckling in the background. Come to think of it, he was starting to feel pretty chipper himself.

14 - THE GROUP

When Tom showed up at Dr. Feelgood's Thursday evening, he heard voices coming from the inner office. "Come on in," Dr. Feelgood called from the back, where he and Tom had their sessions. "Hey, everybody, this is Tom DoRight. Tom, I'd like you to meet Shelly, who has been a patient of mine for the last three months, and Peter, who's been coming here for, what is it, now, six weeks?"

"Yea, going on seven."

"And I'm Carlene," said a dark-haired woman with flashing eyes. "I've been coming for almost a month, and I probably wouldn't be alive today if it weren't for Dr. Feelgood."

"Why's that?" asked Tom.

"Because I didn't know my face from my rear-end before, obviously."

"What?!"

"I had no idea what healthful living was before I developed cancer and was brought to our kind doctor, here. I lived on fast food--Colonel Sanders was my best friend--and drank at least a six-pack of sodas every day, alternating with coffee. If I didn't have my daily chocolate fix I'd kill someone. I was as high-strung as someone could be and still live to talk about it."

"So what do you do now? What have you changed?"

"My weight, to begin with. You should have seen me before. I weighed in today, and I've lost 10 pounds in the last month. No more fried foods right now, although Dr. Feelgood tells me I can eventually have them on occasion--just not now during the intensive healing. I also follow some basic health rules that have made my digestion work for me again."

"Like?"

"Like," Shelly chimed in, "at least 55% of our food has to be high in fiber, from grains like rice or oats, wheat, millet, buckwheat, quinoa or rye, for example."

"Wait a minute," Tom broke in. "I thought we weren't supposed to eat cooked foods."

"Remember, Tom, I told you that not all foods are meant to be eaten raw," interrupted Dr. Feelgood. "Grains are high in fiber, either raw, sprouted or cooked, as long as they are not overcooked to the point that all their nutrients are depleted. You can't eat millet raw, but it still retains its fiber when it's cooked. Of course, so does unbuttered popcorn--as long as it's air-popped. And if peas and beans are not sprouted, then they have to be cooked in order to release the enzymes necessary for their digestion."

"You can eat grains, seeds and nuts in their raw, sprouted state," Shelly added, "but they're also highly nutritious even after they've been cooked. They contain *all* the important nutrients essential for human growth, sustaining health, and preventing disease in perfect combination and balance. Right, doc?"

Dr. Feelgood nodded. "Grains are not only excellent sources of proteins and essential unsaturated fatty acids--which are absolutely necessary for health--they also contain most of the B-complex vitamins, as well as vitamins C, E and A, phosphorus, potassium, calcium, magnesium, selenium and amino acids your body needs."

"Which is why they form the basis for the foods we eat," added Peter.

"I've got one question," Shelly said.

"Just one?" Tom broke in. "I've got a million."

Shelly smiled and went on. "Doc, I'm to the point where I'm afraid to eat anything I used to. I'm afraid that if I put anything in my mouth other than squash or broccoli or brown rice, my whole immune system will fall apart again, and the cancer will come back. I've made such gains already that even my oncologist is getting intrigued and asking for book titles. I don't want to fall back, but occasionally I crave potato chips so much I think I'll lose my mind. I mean, I obsess over them. What can I do? Will it kill me to have a potato chip?"

"No, Shelly," Dr. Feelgood reassured her. "Look, you've done a great job so far of building up your body. You're enormously stronger and more capable of resisting dis-ease now than you were when we first met. You know you can't go back to eating meat every day, like you used to, or toss out all your new-found tofu recipes, or drown yourself in M&Ms. But there's nothing wrong with adding a little variety, a few of your old favorites back into your diet--on a very limited basis. If you've just got to have those potato chips, have some, for heaven's sake! Just don't binge on them. Look for the chips in your natural-foods store that use sea salt, or no salt at all, and have no preservatives. Or try some baked potato chips--that's what I eat, and they're just as tasty as the fried kind, only much better for you."

Peter jumped up. "What about getting off the almond butter, and back to my peanut butter!" he asked indignantly.

Dr. Feelgood laughed so long and loud it brought a smile to everyone's face. "Go ahead," he finally said, wiping his eyes. "Have your peanut butter. You don't even have to buy the health-food-store brand. I've found delicious peanut butter without sugar or preservatives in every supermarket I've checked. It's usually the house brand. They think they're making it cheaper by leaving out the sugar, but they're actually making it healthier! Whatever it takes to let you feel more like a human being again. Just be careful that you don't overdo, like always, because peanut butter does have a lot of fat in it--peanuts are high in fat. That's right, that old word again...."

"Moderation," the group intoned.

Tom took a deep breath. "Doc, I'm glad I'm here. I see why you wanted me to meet some of your other patients. It looks like I may have a future to look forward to after all."

"It's a lot closer than you think, Tom," Carlene spoke up. "I can already feel the changes in my energy. Where I was sleeping twelve hours a day,

I'm now sleeping six, and feeling refreshed. When you do right by your body, it usually does right by you."

"Good words to remember," Shelly added, nodding.

Dr. Feelgood looked at Tom as he spoke to the others in the room. "Tom has always been a man in control, a man of power. He has always liked taking control of everything around him."

"We've all been taking control, since we met Doc Feelgood, by knowing what we're doing every time we put something in our mouths. No more indiscriminate eating for me--or any of us," Peter said, while the others nodded in agreement.

"I've always believed that knowledge is power," Tom said slowly. "I guess I am starting to feel like I'm getting back to the controls."

"Good!" Dr. Feelgood got to his feet. "Thank you all for coming in. I'll see you at your regular appointment times. Go home now, and seize that power!"

For the first time since the pain gripped his chest, Tom knew he was going to be fine.

15 - HEALING FOODS

Tom arranged his notebook on the desk in front of him.

"All set, Master. Teach on."

"Good. It's time to talk about healing foods. Do you have that list of what you ate yesterday that I asked you to keep?" Dr. Feelgood asked.

"Yeah, right here, and I've already started to clean up my act pretty good. See? Instead of pizza, I ordered Chinese last night. Vegetables barely cooked, white rice, egg-drop soup and orange-glazed chicken. Only one concentrated food, with practically raw vegetables--I even got in some of those grains you guys were talking about. Did I do okay?"

"Yes, you did well by having vegetables barely cooked, rather than mushy, the way you used to. Raw is wonderful, too, but I know the taste you were looking for wouldn't have been there raw. But remember, the white rice you ate, which you will typically find in Oriental restaurants, was depleted of

I HAVE A CHOICE?!

fiber and nutrition--it had been polished and bleached, so all the natural minerals are gone. Most Chinese restaurants don't serve brown rice, unfortunately, but if you enjoy eating Chinese food often, you might consider asking the restaurants you patronize to add the choice of brown rice to their menus. Some are actually getting the point and serving brown rice now. And you, my friend, especially for now, would be wise to avoid the white rice at all times, as well as any refined or bleached food devoid of nutrients. Look back over your notes, Tom. It's important for you to stick to the whole grains. Brown rice still has all its nutrients left in it--it doesn't go through a bleaching process, and has probably only had one layer, the outer husk, removed before it reaches you. White rice has had all its fibrous layers removed, then is bleached and polished. Same with your bread--if you eat white bread made with refined, bleached flour, even if the flour has been fortified with vitamins and minerals, it still doesn't have the nutrition you can get from products made with whole, unbleached flour, with natural vitamins and minerals intact."

"Yeah, yeah, I know. Whole wheat bread."

"Back to last night's dinner--you added a protein, the chicken (a concentrated food), to your stomach at the same time as the rice (also a concentrated food). And these two concentrated foods require different enzymes, or digestive juices, for digestion, remember?"

"Oh man--I didn't think about the rice. I thought I was doing so great because I wasn't having potatoes or pasta! Is that why I still got bloated?"

"Probably. Look, Tom, you're working at it, and that's good. The more you learn, the more you'll enjoy working at achieving good health, because you'll start feeling so good, you'll want to maintain that feeling. Believe me, it will become easier. It's like learning a whole new language--but it **has to become a way of life to be beneficial and lasting**. And it has to take place now because of the shape you are currently in."

Dr. Feelgood pointed to Tom's notebook. "I'm going to give you a list of some of the nutritious foods you should rotate around in your diet, along with the in-season fruits we already talked about. Write these down."

- **Brown rice**, especially sweet brown rice. It's more glutinous than most rices, draws toxins out of the colon, and is absolutely necessary during your initial recovery.

- **Miso**, a nutritious soybean paste, is sometimes made with soybeans, rice and/or barley and sea salt, and fermented for either a few months or a few years to develop its rich taste. The versatility of miso is limitless. As a concentrated source of protein and other nutrients, it is also used in place of salt in many instances. The less salty [longer fermented] misos can be used daily to season grains and vegetables, make soup stocks, and add flavor to any food. Macrobiotic diets use miso a great deal. Miso contains enzymes that aid digestion, and like yogurt, it is a living food that contains lactobacillus and other healthful microorganisms. Although there are many varieties available, mugi miso is especially suitable for people with serious illnesses.

- **Shiitake Mushrooms** are good in soups or vegetable dishes. You can get them fresh, or buy them dried and reconstitute with water. They're available almost everywhere these days, but especially in Asian markets. You can also buy them in extract or tincture form at your local health-food store. They'll help you eliminate excess animal fats, and also help to shrink tumors.

- **Seaweed(s) or Sea Vegetables**, especially kombu/kelp and wakame seaweeds, contain a variety of minerals. Wakame is especially high in protein, iron and magnesium, and kombu is especially good for ingesting the fats that clog arteries.

"Slow down, slow down!"
Doc Feelgood waited until Tom looked up from his notebook. "Ready?" Tom nodded.
"Okay, write these down, too:"

Bok choy
Broccoli
Burdock
Radishes
Onions
Garlic
Cauliflower
Carrots

- **Celery**
- **Cabbage**
- **Collard greens**
- **Daikon radish**
- **Brussel Sprouts**
- **Kale**
- **Mustard Greens**
- **Rutabagas**
- **Spinach**
- **Red Potatoes**
- **Squash family, including acorn, buttercup, butternut, hubbard and pumpkin**
- **Soybeans**
- **Tofu**
- **Parsley**
- **Watercress**

Tom groaned. "This diet will turn me into a rabbit!"

"Uh, what's up, doc?" Dr. Feelgood mimicked. "Ever see a sick rabbit? Actually, these are life-giving foods, not empty-calorie foods that carry no nutrition. Our bodies run best on these types of foods."

"Swell. I suppose adding salt is out of the question?"

"Oh, you don't want to do that, Tom."

"I don't?"

"No. Table salt actually leaves harmful deposits in your joints, besides basically throwing your body chemistry out of balance. Instead, let your tongue become accustomed to tasting the natural flavor of food, rather than masking it with table salt or other unnatural seasonings. In your natural-foods stores you will find natural herb-and-spice combinations that are not harmful and are quite delicious. Also, there are the products that taste like soy sauce such as Quick Sip® and Liquid Aminos® that are healthful and enhance the flavors of food that you might consider bland. Spices in moderation are all right, but try to avoid some of the commercial salt combinations, like garlic salt or celery salt, or Italian seasonings with salt as the base. And be especially careful that you avoid MSG--monosodium glutamate. It's very sneaky stuff, and it's in a lot of packaged and canned foods. You've heard people say they're usually hungry an hour or so after they've had Chinese food, right?"

"Well, I know it's a fact, doc. I always order more than I can eat at the table, because I know I'm gonna have another helping before I go to bed that night. Why is it we all feel that way when we eat Chinese?"

"MSG is the culprit. It enhances the flavor, but it also irritates the mucus membrane lining the stomach, leaving you with a feeling that your brain interprets as hunger. MSG can also cause headaches as an allergic reaction and I believe it has been found to cause cancer. Please read the labels of any pre-packaged food you buy, and make sure it doesn't list MSG as one of the ingredients."

"Whoa--it can cause cancer--another possible cause of my problem? Can it also cause diarrhea?"

"Most definitely."

"I guess that explains last night. And I love Chinese!"

"Me, too. You can always ask the chef to not use MSG or sugar. I do. They never seem to mind. So many people today refuse MSG that a lot of places have stopped using it altogether as a matter of course. Besides, all the foods I mentioned a few minutes ago have their own wonderful, aromatic flavors. You can find some great cookbooks in health-food stores or your favorite bookstore that can give you some delicious, live-food-combination ideas. Just use some discretion when you look through them. If their main ingredients are oils, creams, sugars or meats, put the book back on the shelf and look for one that shows a lot of vegetables on the cover."

"I wouldn't even know where to begin with the foods you just mentioned."

"I'll give you a few ideas of what to make with these foods. Yes, it's a different way of eating, but it can also be a delicious way of eating. While you're trying to strengthen your body, get rid of your cancer, and clogged arteries, you're going to need to accept some delicious, new kinds of foods."

Tom forced himself to look at the recipes. They did not look as bad as he was afraid they would.

Nutritious Vegetable Soup
Kombu (seaweed)
Miso paste
1 onion
2-3 Carrots, cut up
2-3 stalks of Celery, cut up
2 medium Red potatoes, cut up
1 clove Garlic

Place several strips of kombu in a container of cold water for an hour until it soaks up the water and at least doubles in size. Fill a 4-5 quart pot half full with filtered water; bring to a boil. Add onions and kombu, let boil for 5 minutes, reduce heat. Add carrots, celery and red potatoes. Simmer 15-20 minutes, remove from heat. Do not over-boil! Immediately add fresh-pressed garlic to taste, using garlic press--a small, inexpensive, hand-held appliance available at any grocery store. Put the clove in the press, and squeeze the garlic out of it into the pot. In a small cup or bowl, add a teaspoon or more (to taste) miso paste to 2-3 tablespoons soup stock; moosh until miso becomes liquidy, then add to the soup and stir. Add more miso or garlic to taste, if necessary. Season with basil, rosemary, cumin, fennel, or other natural herbs and spices. NO SEASONING SALTS. (This recipe combines one concentrated food, with several high-water-content foods. The nutrients remain in the soup even after the vegetables have been cooked, as long as it is not overcooked so all the nutrients are boiled out of it.)

Vegetable Soup Alternatives

1) Replace the red potatoes with sweet brown rice in the above recipe. Wash the rice well, add to boiling water with the onion and kombu; continue with above steps. This makes a thicker soup.
2) Use barley instead of rice or potatoes.
3) Make a nutritious bean soup, adding vegetables after the beans are almost completely cooked. Consult a cookbook for cooking time on each variety of bean you may choose to use.

Broccoli Ideas

Broccoli is an essential cruciferous vegetable, full of vitamins, minerals, and trace elements, and is best eaten raw. Cut florets into bite-size pieces. To cook, steam briefly, or lightly stir-fry in small amount of cold-pressed olive oil, or even a tablespoon of water alone; season with Liquid Aminos® or make a non-dairy dip for the broccoli.

Tofu

Made from soybeans, tofu looks like a white block of curd, and is high in protein, low in unhealthful fats, and delicious in a number of ways. With no real taste of its own, tofu is flavored by what is added to it. Use as a substitute for rice or potatoes in soup, or to replace eggs in many dishes. Tofu comes in firm or soft form. The soft tofu is easily mashed, and can replace eggs, dairy cream or sour cream in many recipes. Firm tofu is better for stir-frying.

Tofu Scrambler

Mash one block of soft tofu, cook in 1 tablespoon cold-pressed olive oil for approx. 2 minutes. Add 1/4 cup water, season with spices and herbs to taste, cook another 2-3 minutes. As an alternative, season with Tofu Scrambler , a boxed mixture available in health-food stores.

Tofu Stirfry

Cut firm tofu block into bite-sized pieces, approx. 1/2" x 1/2" cubed; lightly stirfry in unrefined, toasted sesame oil. Add cut-up broccoli, mustard greens, scallions, and/or parsley. Season with spices, herbs, and 1 tbsp. teriyaki marinade (purchase at natural-food store--check the label--no MSG, remember?) When color of vegetables is brilliant, remove skillet from heat and serve.

Tom looked up. "I don't know, doc. I'm not real big into tofu. Dana has tried to get me to eat it a bunch of times, and I never could stand the taste of it. It's so blah."

"Which essentially means you don't like Dana's cooking," the doctor replied. "Frankly, tofu has no taste of its own. If you didn't like Dana's recipes, perhaps she was using some kind of spice or herb that doesn't appeal to you. Experiment. You'll find there are a lot of possibilities with this particular food. It's extremely versatile. Your best bet would be to look for combinations and recipes in a cookbook that doesn't promote lard and the like--or, better yet, maybe you can take a class in macrobiotic cooking. Check around. I'm sure you can find a healthful cooking class. Get to know your local health-food-store owners--they're the ones who usually know where things are happening. You might even meet some interesting new significant

I HAVE A CHOICE?!   109

other who can share the cooking with you. Certainly, you'll meet like-minded people--like Shelly and Peter and Carlene--and you can learn about their recipes and successes, too. It's very beneficial for the healing process. Of course, if you're too busy to cook or take classes, there are places that will prepare and deliver healthy meals to you anywhere you'd like."

"You mean like Paul and Linda McCartney usually order? I thought that was all specially prepared just for them."

"No. Those places that deliver to them will deliver for anybody--even us simple folk."

Tom chuckled. "Listen, speaking of Shelly and Carlene--not that I'm referring to them as 'simple folk'--are they both married?"

Dr. Feelgood chuckled back. "Shelly is, I'm afraid--very married, in fact. But Carlene isn't."

"Really? I would have thought the other way... Listen, I don't suppose you'd give me Carlene's number..."

"No, but I can tell you she goes to the same yoga class Dana goes to."

"Hey, Dana's been pushing me to go with her to that tonight! Are you sure she'll be there?"

"It's worth a try, isn't it? While you're there, why don't you ask her about some of the books she's read. She's really getting to be very well-versed in healthy foods and cooking."

"Sounds like a plan, doc. Sounds like a plan."

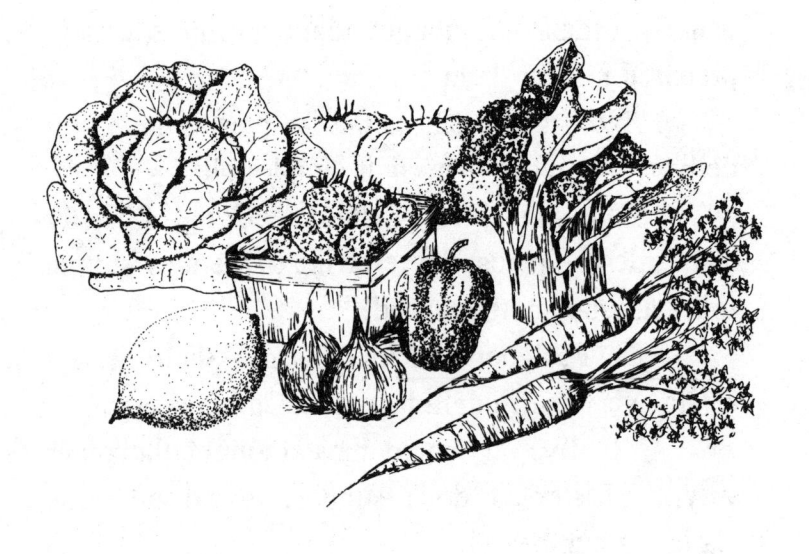

16 - DESTRUCTIVE FOODS

"Well, doc, before I get too excited about tonight, I know you've got more bad news for me. You asked for questions. What else do I have to avoid, and for how long do I have to avoid it?"

"Like I said, while you are healing, you need to avoid stress. Lay off refined and high-fat foods. Avoid being sedentary, smoking cigarettes, drinking alcohol--and any other pollutants you indulge in. If you're talking about foods..."

"You know I am, doc!"

"Okay, avoid ALL refined foods of any kind. And stay away from anything that contains table salt, white sugar, white flour, caffeine (that's coffee, black tea and chocolate, in that order), red meat, eggs and dairy products. God isn't cruel, though. You can still enjoy a large number of alternatives to these things--if you'll give them a try. It's just that some things are an acquired taste. To replace table salt, for example, turn either to miso or seaweed for a natural, salty flavor. You can also use a limited amount of sea salt, which is less processed, and non-iodized (doesn't have sodium iodide or potassium iodide added to it). Instead of white sugar, try organic **unfiltered honey** on occasion, organic **brown-rice syrup**, or a pure cane product, such as '**Sucanat®**.'"

"Sucanat? What's that? It sounds like some kind of nutmeat."

"Actually, the name is a shortened version of 'Sugar Cane Natural.' Su-ca-nat, see? It's sugar cane that's simply been ground up instead of bleached or processed. It looks kind of like brown sugar, but instead of being processed white sugar with added molasses, it has all the natural cane still in it."

"Maybe I'm sick, but that actually sounds kinda good."

Dr. Feelgood laughed. "Oh, it is. But for the time being, while you are healing your body, you would really do best to avoid sweets altogether. Cancer feeds off sugar. Even fruits that are very high in sugar, such as dates or bananas, are not as good to eat right now as the low-sugar-content ones. When I say avoid sugar right now, I mean it. Cancer loves it."

"Unfortunately, so do I."

"Well, Tom, we've got to starve your cancer,

not feed it. Giving in to the temptation of a doughnut or coffee isn't just about your weight or nerves right now. We're talking about your life. To replace white flour and the breads, pastas and pastries made with it, try foods made with **whole-grain flours**. They're much healthier, they have a nuttier flavor, and they're actually lighter in your body, because they won't simply sit in your intestines and make you feel sluggish. You can even get pasta made from Jerusalem artichokes. It's the best spaghetti, fettucini, and lasagna you've ever tasted--and it doesn't get as sticky in the pot, or in your gut!"

Tom looked relieved. "I love pasta!"

"I know. You don't have to give it up, you just have to modify your shopping habits a little."

"Okay, good. What else? How can I replace my chocolate?"

"First, let's talk about caffeine. Caffeine overloads your adrenal glands, which, in turn, breaks down your immune system. Switch to non-caffeinated drinks, especially **carob-roasted beverages, roasted-grain beverages,** and **herb teas**--some of which are very good for you. They all taste delicious on their own."

"What about decaf coffee?"

"I'd drink it sparingly, to be honest. Unless it's

been decaffeinated via a healthy water process, it can end up being as bad for you as regular coffee--less caffeine, but lots of oils and chemicals."

"Great. So how do I wake up in the morning?"

"Try ginseng or pau d'arco teas. They have similar qualities to caffeinated drinks, but without the heart-shocking aspects. You can also look for a specific brand, called Sports Tea®, which is both refreshing and stimulating, yet has no caffeine or harmful chemicals in it."

"Where can I find that? No, don't tell me--at my local health-food store, right?"

"Or at some health-oriented restaurants, or even in some chain supermarkets."

"But what about my chocolate?"

"Try carob."

"I hate carob."

"Chocolate is a problem. We both know it. There is no easy answer. Besides, you can't eat chocolate without sugar in it, because it's very bitter in its natural state."

"So, you mean...."

"That's right. During your recovery, the only thing you can do is apply a little self-discipline."

"I hate that."

"I don't blame you. But it's better than

surgery."

"Tell me, doc, that I'll be able to eat it again someday."

"You'll be able to eat it again someday."

"For real?"

"For real. But not during recovery. And not as a steady diet."

Tom made a disgusted face. "Well, then, have you at least got anything in your little black bag to replace my craving for meat that won't bring on visions of factories?"

"Of course! Look for alternate products, such as pre-formed burgers or sausages made from tofu, or vegetables and grains. Check the labels, though--don't buy any vegetarian junk-food. Just because it has no meat doesn't mean it has no junk. You can tell what's good and what's not by the ingredients. A good rule of thumb is simple word recognition. If it's a food ingredient, it will say something like 'wheat,' or 'soybeans.' If you can't pronounce it, or get a mental image of it on your plate, it's probably a chemical. Avoid all chemicals. And remember, if it's got MSG in it, put it back on the shelf."

"What about preservatives?"

"**Especially** preservatives. And remember,

sugar and salt are natural preservatives--so the less the better. You can still eat the skinless, white meat of fowl very occasionally--just try to avoid the ones from the supermarket, because most of those are raised in such unhealthy conditions."

"Yeah, I remember."

"Again, check a natural-foods market if you feel you must have some chicken or turkey, but remember--no red meat for now.

"So bacon and eggs are definitely out."

"I'd like to say they aren't, but they are. Yes, you can find turkey bacon, and even vegetarian bacon-like strips, but they're so loaded down with fats and preservatives that I can't recommend them. Later on, down the line, when you're strong enough for a little variety, maybe--now and then, not as a steady diet. But as far as eggs are concerned, tofu makes a wonderful substitute. I'd like you to avoid the egg-replacement products since they're essentially chemical compounds, but you can always eat just egg whites, and leave the fat-laden yolks out."

"Like just the whites of a hard-boiled egg?"

"Right. Or separate the yolk and scramble the whites with some veggies and herbs. Delicious."

"And the dairy product replacements..." Tom started flipping back through his notes.

"...are soy cheese, soy milks, rice milks, nut milks and soy, rice and nut ice creams," the doctor filled in. "They won't cause mucus formation, and are as delicious as regular cheese, ice cream or milk. I personally cannot tell them apart, except after I eat them--I don't get an allergic reaction."

"You know, all this sounds awfully familiar. I know my gastroenterologist friend, Don Belcher, wanted me to cut out a lot of garbage, as he called it, and eat more veggies. He just never explained it the way you have. I don't know why--somehow, it seems easier this way."

"Well, Tom, you weren't ready to hear him before. And, as you say, knowledge is power."

"And having it imposed is not the same as choosing it on your own," Tom continued for him.

"Right. Macrobiotic diets, which use a lot of these foods we're talking about, have turned around a lot of illness--when the patient adhered to the diet during the cancer-elimination process, and when the necessary aspects that go along with the healing were in place."

"Meaning?"

"For one thing, you've got to have a positive attitude--you've got to believe in the form of treatment you're undergoing for it to be successful.

For another thing, treatment will have a far better chance of success if started soon after detection. And the type of illness or cancer being treated is always another consideration."

Tom smiled confidently. "You know, doc, I feel good about all this. Really good."

"Good! Then before you leave for today, let's talk about another really important thing you put into your body--fluids."

17 - LIQUIDS & JUICING

"Are you talking about water?" Tom asked after he had gotten himself resettled with his notebook.

Dr. Feelgood nodded. "Definitely water. And juices--fresh, raw juices. But let's start with water. How much of it do you drink every day?"

"Enough. A couple of glasses every day at least."

"Bottled or tap?"

"Tap. I don't drink enough to buy bottled water, and I'm not into fads."

"It's not a fad, Tom. You should avoid tap water in just about any town in America. Our water contains a lot of chemicals and inorganic minerals harmful to human health, as well as viruses, and microbes that are deadly...I could go on and on about tap water."

"Microbes? I've heard that word, but what's the definition?"

"Microbes are microscopic organisms that are

unable to be detected without a microscope, specifically germs or bacteria that undermine the immune systems of humans when they enter the digestive tract. Didn't you see the reports on the news the other night about the thousands of people who've been drinking tap water that are becoming sick, and hundreds of them have died recently--all of their deaths have been linked to the microbes in the tap water they were drinking."

"I did see that report. But I thought it was just in the midwest area, wasn't it?"

"No, Tom, they said in the report that it has been found in the tap water all over the United States, now, including California and New York. Drink filtered or bottled water, both of which remove many of these harmful microbes and chemicals. In some areas, tap water has even been known to cause sterility in women--not that you need to worry about that. But you don't need all the chemicals and other possible deadly things it contains. However, you do need to drink a lot more water and a lot less carbonated sodas and coffee. For one thing, you don't need the stimulants. For another, your heart and colon need some pampering and stimulating of a different kind, such as what you get with juicing and herbs."

"You mean squeezing oranges for juice? My ex-girlfriend bought me an orange juicer, but she took it back when we broke up."

"So you've actually done fresh fruit juicing? That's good. Now let's talk about extracting juice from vegetables. I want you to start juicing for health."

"Like making my own V-8?"

"Yes and no. We're talking about a lot of the same vegetables along with some others, in different mixtures. The real difference, though, is in making and drinking them fresh, rather than buying the canned stuff. Canned vegetables have been cooked way past 120°F, which, you'll remember, kills off their enzyme integrity. Only fresh, uncooked vegetables and fruits retain their enzymes and natural oxygen. Raw, naturally-pressed fruit juices have wonderful blood-cleansing and revitalizing capabilities, because they have a high hydrogen peroxide H_2O_2 content, which kills off harmful bacteria and microbes. Fresh vegetable juices also contain large amounts of H_2O_2, and are excellent for rebuilding muscles, and returning a body to health. I highly recommend juicing therapy, especially now, when you need to cleanse and rebuild your entire system."

"What I really want to clean out is the cancer."

"And that's just what you'll do. Juices, with all their wonderful, active, complex-substance enzymes, are so powerful they can actually digest cancers--not if you continue to eat a high-fat diet full of processed foods at the same time, of course. A weakened body simply cannot fight off the continued abuse. But if you drink raw juices while you're cleaning out your toxins and building up your immune system with the proper nutrition, you have a better than good chance of destroying that disease-friendly environment, and ridding your body of all cancerous growth."

"Geez, I just can't believe we were never taught this in school. Even today! Last night my son came over--he goes to USC--and we talked about this stuff. He didn't have a clue about any of it. Isn't this more important than calculus?"

Dr. Feelgood shook his head ruefully. "Yes, of course. We should be teaching our children the nutritional basics, right along with the facts of life, so they can learn to live healthy lives--but just look at how much controversy there is about basic sex-and-drug education that could help keep our kids from killing themselves! Getting this kind of 'radical' nutritional information into the mainstream school system is proving to be an uphill battle--although trust me, there are a lot of people working on it. You can help by asking your son to petition to make nutrition classes part of the general education curriculum in college; every little bit helps. But the reality is that much of what keeps the world going is business, and business today is primarily concerned with the bottom line, not the public's health. Like I said the other day, we get more of our 'education' from advertising than facts, and have ever since TV was born. What's worse, we've been taught--and are teaching our kids--to be victims."

"Hey, careful, doc!" Tom blistered. "I'm no victim--and anybody who tries to make me into one had better watch out!"

"Well, maybe you're not, in the sense you're thinking of- -but consider this. What's your first response when you don't feel good? To call a doctor, right?"

"Yeah, of course. What else?"

"When you got sick, did it occur to you to do some research, and at least go in to see your medical professional knowing what you needed to tell him, what kinds of answers he needed to his questions?"

Tom started to form an angry answer, then stopped. He was quiet for a few seconds, then said, "No, that never occurred to me."

"Did you ever consider that maybe you were responsible for your problems? And that maybe you could heal them? Heal them without a third party--someone theoretically wiser and more highly trained, but who does not live inside your skin, and, therefore, does not really know what you are doing, feeling, or sensing. Yet you have in the past allowed that third party to take charge and attempt to fix you."

Tom swallowed. "And if that third party doesn't ask the right questions, or I don't give the right answers so he understands them, or worse, he just simply goofs...I get your point. I guess I am setting myself up to be a victim. Damn! I never thought of it that way before!"

"Well, don't feel too bad," Dr. Feelgood smiled. "Most of us don't. That's why education is so very important. When we don't teach our kids what can go wrong, and how they can avoid it, we set them up to be victims. When we don't teach low-income women how to prevent unwanted pregnancies, we set them up to be victims. When we don't...."

"Doc! Doc!"

Dr. Feelgood took a deep breath. "Sorry, another one of my pet bandwagons. The idea is, we need to go back to being old-fashioned Americans, the kind who rolled up their sleeves and took care of themselves--independent, self-sufficient, and even somewhat self-educated. We need to take responsibility for our own lives, so no one else can victimize us again when it comes to our own bodies."

"And that means drinking fresh vegetable juice?"

Dr. Feelgood laughed. "Well, that's part of it."

"One thing I don't get, though. Why just drink the juice? Shouldn't I eat the whole vegetable? I thought you said veggies were full of fiber, and fiber is like an intestinal broom."

"Good question. Again the answer is yes, and no. Your body is in a weakened state right now. Removing the fiber from the fruits and 'veggies,' as you call them, lets your body digest and assimilate the nutrients from the juice very quickly, with a minimum of effort and exertion on the part of your digestive system. Remember, fruit juices are the cleansers of the human system, vegetable juices the builders and regenerators. You could actually live on juices for a period of time if you were ever so inclined--don't worry, I'm not asking you to do that! The look on your face...! However, fresh, raw, unpreserved juices do contain all the amino acids, minerals, salts, enzymes and vitamins you body needs to nourish and regenerate your cells, tissues, glands and organs with a minimum of digestive effort."

"Okay, so what do I drink? Just any old juice? I kinda like tomato juice."

"Let's start with carrot juice as the base of your vegetable juicing combinations. It will clear out all the mucus built up in your body, which will help you start dropping those unwanted pounds, and take some of the strain off your heart and lower back. Carrot juice is the total opposite of cows' milk, which builds mucus up in the system, remember? Oh, one other important point: a lot of the sprays we use today to get rid of bugs on our fruits and vegetables are toxic..."

"Tell me about it! At least I've read about pesticides in the papers, and heard about them on the news. That's why I asked you earlier if it was safe to eat raw foods since you don't know what's still on them."

"Right. Organically grown foods are certainly safer to eat than commercially grown foods. But the toxins from the pesticides are retained in the fiber of the produce, so it's not a problem in the fiber-free juice."

"That's a relief! Okay, so can I make the

juices with my blender?"

"No, you'll need to buy a juice extractor. They come in all price ranges, from as low as $30 to as high as $2,000. I wouldn't bother with a $30 juicer, though."

"In other words, you get what you pay for?"

"Precisely. It would probably break down on you just as you were getting into the swing of things--not a strong enough motor. I've seen some good juice extractors in the $70 range that last for two or three years of fairly constant use. You can always get a more elaborate one later on, if you decide to continue juicing after your recovery."

"Why would I want to do that?!"

"Possibly because you've learned to love it. Many people do. There is nothing quite like fresh, vital juice in the morning, or as a mid-day pick-me-up. For right now, though, I suggest you get a moderately-priced juicer."

"I would swear I have something that says 'juice extractor' in a box in the back of my closet."

"I believe every household should have one out on the counter--not hidden in a closet--for constant use. By the way, there are wonderful books on what juice combinations are good for what disorder--even baldness! Look in..."

"I know, I know--my local health-food store."

"Right! <u>And</u> in many bookstores. They'll give you some ideas for experimenting. In the meantime, plan to use:

> **Carrots** (powerful blood cleanser/muscle builder)
> **Beets** (powerful blood cleanser)
> **Spinach** (powerful blood cleanser)
> **Celery** (contains high amount of vital organic sodium)
> **Garlic** (especially good for your heart)

"There are a lot of other vegetables you can juice together, and we'll work with them as well. But these are the basics..."

"Did I hear you say 'garlic?'"

"Yes. Not only is it a wonderful heart strengthener and toner, it's also very mellow when you combine it with carrot and beet juice--many people who don't like carrot juice alone love it with garlic. You'll see. Some other good combinations are:

Carrot, beet, cucumber
Carrot, beet, parsley, cucumber
Carrot, potato, parsley, lettuce
Carrot, spinach
Carrot, spinach, beet
Carrot, celery, cucumber
Carrot, celery, parsley, beet
Carrot, beet, cucumber, parsley, garlic

"These can be altered to taste as you start experimenting, but you'll want to use approximately 10 carrots to 1/2 a beet or cucumber, or 2 stalks of celery, or 1 clove of garlic, etc. Never use equal combinations of carrot to beet or any other vegetable, because carrots are easy to drink straight, but not all the others are. You can only drink about an ounce of straight beet juice, for example, before you start getting dizzy, because its purifying abilities go to work in your blood so fast. It's very concentrated. You really need carrot as your main juice. I'm sure if you play around with it a bit, you can have fun while you're getting healthy."

"How much should I drink at a time?" Tom asked as he made notes. "How much per day? And should I drink it every day, or every other day, or what?"

"For now I'd like to see you juice daily. To start, drink at least eight ounces of a carrot-juice combination, such as carrot, beet, ginger and garlic. The ginger is good for improving your digestion; the carrot, of course, will eliminate the mucus from your body and help you lose weight; the beet will purify your blood; and the garlic will purify your blood and also help strengthen your heart. As soon as you can, work up to a quart every day for at least two months, with a few days off here and there during that time, especially since you're working to clear up such serious conditions as cancer and heart disease. Your skin may turn slightly yellow, but this effect is harmless and temporary, and merely indicates that your body (especially your liver) is being cleansed, purified and strengthened that much more quickly."

"A quart--that's like two pints, right? Or, say, four cups of coffee?"

"Volume-wise, it's just about exactly that. There are two cups to the pint, two pints to the quart, and most people drink a little more than an actual cup when they have coffee."

"No sweat. I do four cups before the first scene is set up. So I drink veggies instead of coffee. All I really care about is that I've got something to drink. Is it okay if I juice in the morning, and take it with me in a thermos?"

"Absolutely fine. Just don't let it sit too long without refrigeration. And make sure the juice is kept cold in a glass-lined thermos, not an aluminum one."

"No problem. Thank heavens! Something on this regimen I can do easily! Now all I've got to do is get a juicer--no, wait--I'm sure I've got one. Dana gave it to me last Christmas. I put it in the back of the closet with all her other weird gifts. I guess I'll drag it out and put it to work. Hey, maybe I could ask Carlene over to get juiced!"

18- GRASSES & CLEANSING

Tom started to close his notebook, but Dr. Feelgood shook his head. "Vegetables and fruits aren't the only juices I want to talk to you about. **Green Grasses** are in a category unto themselves."

"Now you're kidding, aren't you, Doc? Grass is for cattle and goats!"

"This is for real. Grass is the only vegetation on this entire planet that can give sole nutritional support to the human body from birth to old age. The most common grasses we use in this country are alfalfa, barley and wheatgrass. The power of the juice from these grasses (especially wheatgrass) comes from the effectiveness of chlorophyll. Chlorophyll has a molecular structure almost identical to hemoglobin (the protein of red-blood cells), but it contains an atom of iron, while blood has an atom of magnesium. Fresh wheatgrass juice, therefore, can literally clean out your blood. Large amounts of it act just like a blood transfusion. And

I HAVE A CHOICE?!

chlorophyll is very high in oxygen, which, as you recall, is important."

"Right, because cancer is anaerobic and cannot exist in the presence of pure oxygen," Tom recited from memory.

"Exactly. Excellent. Have you ever noticed, Tom, that when an animal gets sick, it instinctively knows to eat grass? Animals will feed exclusively on grasses and green leaves when they have an internal disturbance, until they feel well again. This allows them to eliminate their bodies of toxins immediately (often by throwing up the contents of their stomach), plus they get all their nutritional requirements while their bodies become detoxified and balanced."

"Lovely picture."

"That's nature, Tom. Now, wheatgrass juice is the richest nutritional liquid known to man. It contains the greatest variety of minerals, vitamins, and trace elements of all vegetables. Fifteen pounds of fresh wheatgrass are equal in nutritional value to 350 pounds of the most choice vegetables. It is probably one of the most effective known treatments against cancerous growths."

"Kills cancer," Tom read aloud as he wrote. "Juice and drink by the buckets."

Dr. Feelgood chuckled. "Do that and you'll

quickly be nauseous. Too much at first will free up all the free radicals and toxins in your body and make you avoid it altogether. I wouldn't want to see you lose all those wonderful benefits by overdoing a good thing. By the way, you can find several books out on the market now about wheatgrass juice and wheatgrass therapy. One of my favorites is *How I Conquered Cancer Naturally*, by Edie Mae. It's a story about her overcoming the odds when conventional doctors told her it was impossible for her to live if she didn't follow their advice. She opted not to be cut up, piece by piece, and instead found the miracle sprouts, live foods and wheatgrass juice, which saved her life. Wheatgrass therapy has led the way to complete cures for both AIDS and cancer patients who started treatment early after detection."

"AIDS? I'll bet that's what Jason did, huh? God, if only Greg had known about this stuff.... How long before you see any difference?"

"Dramatic results usually show up in a matter of weeks. I can recommend several clinics where you can receive this therapy if you want to take a vacation. Or you can do it at home, either buying large amounts of wheatgrass juice from your local health-food store, or growing and juicing your own. You'll need a wheatgrass juicer if you want to do it yourself. You have to drink it fresh every day--it can't sit around for more than a few hours before the enzymes lose their potency."

"Isn't there any other way to get the stuff down? The idea of drinking grass is a little tough for me."

"I take alfalfa tabs every day to make sure I'm getting enough chlorophyll. You can get wheatgrass or barley grass in tabs or capsules, too, but during recovery, I would really advise you to drink the juice."

"Geez. With all this stuff, I'll really get cleaned out!"

"Well, yes and no."

"Again with the yes and no?"

"You wouldn't want to start a deep body cleansing or even a fast without making sure the toxins you were trying to flush weren't, instead, being re-absorbed."

"Well, that makes sense. How would I take care of that?"

"You'd need to take regular colonics and/or enemas to help clean out your intestines and colon, so the waste matter would be flushed out of your body, rather than be absorbed right back into your cleaned-out bloodstream."

Tom put down his pen, and gave the doctor a rueful look. "I hate enemas."

"Did I give you the impression I like them? They aren't something anybody would love doing, but, frankly, they are necessary. For deeper cleansing, though, enemas alone just aren't enough. Waste matter finds its way into pockets in the small intestine, and can sit there for years without moving on through the large intestine and out of the body. Over time, it putrefies and builds up more and more bacteria. If you're doing a deep cleansing and you don't remove this matter from the intestine and colon physically, either through a colonic or an enema, it can get loosened and re-absorbed back into your bloodstream, which would make your own blood even more toxic."

"How do you give yourself a colonic?"

"You don't. And you shouldn't try to do a really deep cleansing by yourself. You can, of course, but generally, the best approach is to go to a clinic. You can go for one treatment, or for two or three each week for a couple of weeks. There are a number of them around that are very reasonably priced. Most people on a deep cleansing go to a clinic for the treatment."

"Sorry, but I really don't look forward to that."

"I've had many patients who felt the same way before they had a colonic. Afterward, they said their energy level was so wonderful and they felt so light, they couldn't wait to go back for another. Colonics can also help if you suffer from headaches, because they release the buildup of pressure from toxins in your bloodstream. Usually, they are given in a series of 3-6 treatments, over a two-or-more-weeks period."

"Are they absolutely necessary?"

"If you were going on a fast, absolutely yes. During a gentle cleansing, like the one you're undertaking, they're not as critical. A fast is the quickest way to clean out a body, and, therefore, the quickest way to reintroduce toxins into the bloodstream. Usually, when someone goes on a fast, he or she only takes in filtered waters, herb teas, and possibly fruit and vegetable juices--no food that has to be chewed. This way, the body can use its energy in the cleansing process, not the digestion process."

"Are you going to make me go on a fast?"

"I'm not going to make you do anything. I'm going to make certain recommendations..."

"Yeah, yeah, I know, it's my choice what I do. So, do you recommend that I go on a fast?"

"Not immediately. Even though it would speed up the rejuvenation process of your body since the cleansing is so much quicker, I'd rather get your body strong first, and get you used to this new way of thinking about food as fuel, rather than simple tongue pleasure. I must warn you about something, though." Dr. Feelgood's tone suddenly changed. "Getting healthy is somewhat addictive. As you start to feel better, you're going to want to do more to feel even better still. This is one of those areas where it's easy to become radical. Please, Tom, whenever you decide you are ready to go on a fast, don't try it without supervision. I'd want to monitor you very closely during that time. I want your promise on that."

"Geez, Doc, I can't imagine wanting to do it in the first place, but okay, you've got my promise." Tom smiled as he mocked writing in his notebook. "No fasting without supervision. Well, I don't think you need to worry. The thought of not having anything to eat so that putrefied gunk can get into my bloodstream just makes me want to heave."

"How delicately you state things, Tom. Listen, before you go, there's a special program I'd like you to watch tonight on alternative healing--the previews look good. In the past many of these so-called educational shows have turned out to be such big disappointments, like some show that covered homeopathy last year, and managed to discount everything positive."

"Yeah, I know the show you're talking about--30/30, right? I don't think you have to worry about the one tonight. I already knew about it, because my buddy Gil called to tell me about it. I don't usually watch his stuff, because then I'd lose my last excuse not to hire the guy. I really like him, but I've never been really impressed with his work. If you say it's important, though, I'll try to force myself to watch."

Dr. Feelgood laughed. "I appreciate it, especially since it's obviously going to cause you so much discomfort. Hopefully, you'll learn enough to compensate for the pain."

Tom laughed, too. "Aw, what the hell. Gil's got some heart problems too, but he's been playing tennis every day again, and he says he's feeling great. Maybe they'll talk about what he's doing. He's so damn closed-mouthed--I asked him once what kind of voodoo medicine he was taking, but he wouldn't tell me."

"Well, if you asked him that way, can you blame him?"

"Huh. Probably not. Anything special you want me to watch for?"

"I don't know what the show is going to cover. Just watch it, and we'll talk about it at your next session."

19 - HOMEOPATHY

"Hey, doc," Tom started, as he walked into the office. "Did you watch the other night? *Secrets of Alternative Healing*--what an eye-opener!"

"I'm glad you watched it, Tom. I thought it was wonderful to have two hours of prime-time, major-network focus on alternative healing. They brought out a lot of great facts. And I'm glad they spent so much time talking about cayenne. I can't say enough about that wonderful herb. It heals in so many ways."

"I talked to Gil after the show. He says that's what he takes every day for his heart--that and cactus. Geez, cayenne sounds like a wonder drug all by itself. I didn't even know it could improve circulation, much less all the other things it does. My sister had a uterine fibroid tumor, and had to have a hysterectomy just like the woman on the show almost did. I'll bet if she had known cayenne could shrink the tumor, she would have opted to take a pepper capsule four times a day before she just agreed to the surgery."

Dr. Feelgood nodded. "And it might have worked for her, too. I've heard of it working like this in many instances. Unfortunately, you can't always be guaranteed results as quickly, or even the same, as the woman on the show last night."

"Yeah, but it would have been nice if she'd had the option at least to try it first."

"That's what we're working to achieve, my friend. Hopefully, last night's program will help to do just that. All we can do is try to make as many people as possible aware that they have choices in their health care."

"You know what part I found really fascinating, doc?"

The doctor raised his eyebrows at Tom's slightly accusatory tone. "The camera angles?" he asked lightly.

"Very funny. I was talking about the part on homeopathy. You know about that stuff, don't you?"

"Most definitely. And I take it you'd like to talk about it today?"

"Well, yeah. I was wondering when you were going to bring it up, since it seems to be so important. Dana--and Carlene--keep telling me to ask, but I kept

I HAVE A CHOICE?!

saying, 'Hey, he'll get to it when he's ready.' So are you ready yet?"

Dr. Feelgood's belly laugh echoed around the room.

"Okay, okay," Tom said after a minute, somewhat sheepishly. "I guess I deserve that. I was probably too closed-minded to be ready for it before."

The doctor wiped his eyes. "Oh, Tom, you're really wonderful. I'm so glad that show was on last night!"

"Gee, doc, I'm glad I can provide such great entertainment for you," Tom said wryly.

The doctor settled back into his chair. "Well, Tom, where would you like to start?"

"Okay, how about with what they said last night--that some really bad chronic conditions can be cured by homeopathy, not just symptomatically suppressed. Like that guy with the severe allergy to sage who had such bad asthma? He said after just one year he was completely cured of his asthma, and cured of some other lousy habits at the same time, because he and his homeopath worked on his entire constitution, not just his nose. Before I met you, I'd never met a doctor--even friends of mine--who had more than a few minutes for me and my questions in the office. This doctor spent two hours with the guy, and found out everything about him--even what he likes to eat."

"Right. That was the 'taking of the case,' as they say in classical homeopathy. Did you catch the part where they said the patient is treated on three levels?"

"Uh, yeah--physical, mental and emotional, right?"

"Exactly."

"I liked what they said about the plagues--you know, the ones that had ravaged Europe since the dawn of civilization--and how no medicine had a truly positive effect until homeopathy."

"That's true, too. You can look it up in the history books--if you can find an old medical book of the times."

"It's such fascinating stuff!" Dr. Feelgood smiled as Tom jumped up excitedly. "Like that Sam HomeRun guy. Here he's perfectly healthy, and he takes some Peruvian bark, and he gets the chills and fevers, just like as if he has malaria. So he dilutes the bark a bunch of times, and each time, it becomes less toxic, until finally it's diluted so much it isn't toxic at all. So then he gives the diluted stuff to some people who already have malaria, and it gets rid of their chills and fever! The very symptoms the undiluted bark had given him. Geez! It's incredible. Who would of thought of that? I would never have thought of that! And it worked! That's what we were getting so excited about when we watched the show, doc. I mean, the idea really works."

"We? You watched the show with a friend? Gee, Tom, that friend wouldn't happen to be Carlene, would it?"

Tom grinned. "Now, Doc, you know I can't tell you that! Patient privilege and all...."

Dr. Feelgood grinned back. "Well, in any case, I'm glad homeopathy excites you, because, yes, I was going to bring it up--it is important. Let's get down to the lesson."

Tom opened his notebook. "Ready!"

"Homeopathy is a form of healing that deals strictly with the body's vital force, or enzyme activity. Its systematic approach was developed by German physician Samuel Hahnemann--not HomeRun--back in the late 18th century, but homeopathy's basic fundamentals have been known and used by physicians for at least 2300 years. In the 4th century B.C., a Greek physician wrote, 'Through the like, disease is produced, and through the application of the like it is cured.' Hahnemann popularized the phrase 'similia similibus curentur,' which means 'like is cured by like.'"

"Like malaria-producing stuff curing malaria?"

"Exactly. Suppose you had a snake bite--what do you think you would be given as an antidote?"

"Snake venom, right?"

"Right. To counteract the bite, you take a minute dose of the correct venom. It works just as you described with the malaria: if you have a perfectly healthy body, and give it a homeopathic remedy that causes, for example, heart palpitations, that body would experience heart palpitations. But, if you gave that same remedy to a person who already had heart palpitations, the symptoms would be relieved, and the actual condition alleviated. According to Samuel Hahnemann, 'A substance which produces symptoms in a healthy person cures those same symptoms in a sick person.' And the doses given are so minute, they don't overpower a body, like drugs can."

"One thing I'm not clear on--I may have gone to the john during this part--how do you take these remedies? By shot? I gotta be honest; I hate shots almost as much as I hate knives."

"No, no, relax. It's not by shot. Most homeopathic remedies come in a milk-sugar formula in the form of either pellets or tablets that dissolve under your tongue, or in dilutions preserved in alcohol."

"That I can handle. Especially the alcohol part."

"Ha ha. By the way, not to get on another political harangue, but did you know that homeopathy is practiced in England, France, Germany, Israel, Italy, Greece, Russia, Mexico, Brazil, Argentina, South Africa and India, just to name a few countries? It's considered an integral part of 'conventional' medicine in most of these places, all of which have numerous homeopathic medical universities. At the beginning of the 20th century, in fact, we had several homeopathic medical schools here in the U.S., too. Today, we don't have any."

"Why? What happened? Why don't we recognize it like the other countries, if it's so effective, and obviously logical? I mean, geez, they said the British Royal Family has been using it continually for the last 150 years, and at least half of British physicians recommend homeopathic treatment for their patients."

"There are a number of reasons, but the primary one is that the American medical community has worked so hard to eliminate this type of treatment. Part of the problem has been that researchers can't provide the kind of evidence to back up their results that the scientific community considers valid. Another factor is that the profits in homeopathy are so much lower than for 'traditional' treatments. And, quite frankly, doctors being educated today are taught that homeopathy is absolutely ineffective 'hocus pocus,' despite all the documented proof that it works and has no ill side effects. Nowadays, most M.D.s have very little control over their practices. Drug and insurance companies don't allow them much creative freedom. Of course, neither does the average American, with his demands for a quick fix, however costly or painful, rather than permanent relief down the road."

Tom shook his head. "I'm not taking on the guilt, it's anti-constructive--my doctor told me so." He grinned, and Dr. Feelgood grinned back. "But it doesn't seem fair that it's so difficult to get this information and treatment, when so many of us desperately need it. Especially the information. Like, isn't there a homeopathic cancer pill I can take to get rid of my cancer?"

"Not exactly, but kind of."

"Another yes and no."

"Another yes and no. You see, homeopathy

works on a micro-nutritional basis. Minute doses of a remedy, sometimes diluted to the point where only the essence, or the molecular blueprint, of the remedy remains, stimulate the body's natural defense system against the given malady, which, in turn, fights it off with this immune-system boost. Your homeopathic doctor may not always find the exact right remedy for you immediately, because your healing depends on your body's basic constitution, and sometimes, the first remedy chosen for you won't work."

"Yeah, well, what else is new? Do you have any idea how many times I've been given a prescription to 'try?' The latest 'experimental' drug...."

"The 'ole guinea-pig medicine?' That's what one of my patients calls it. Well, there are valid reasons for such trial-and error, believe it or not, but let's not get sidetracked into that. In homeopathy, if you don't notice a change soon after starting a remedy, it could be because you are not taking it on schedule as you are supposed to, or it could be the wrong remedy. In that case, a new remedy may make all the difference in the world. It works through simple trial and error."

"So you have to experiment, just like with drugs?"

"Yes and no."

Tom moaned, and Dr. Feelgood smiled.

"Yes, you have to do some experimentation, but no, homeopathic remedies are nothing like drugs. Most conventional drugs work to suppress symptoms. With homeopathy, the body strengthens itself while working to eliminate the cause, rather than just the symptoms, of the dis-ease. Eliminating the cause, of course, will also eliminate the symptoms associated with the cause--but not immediately. In fact, you may feel worse before you begin to feel better, because you are alleviating the dis-ease or disorder from the inside out."

"Like my laundry comes out when I do it myself?"

Dr. Feelgood grinned and shook his head. "Let's say you have something attacking a vital organ. That organ, during the healing process, will be healed before any other part of the body. In homeopathy, the body is healed from the top to the bottom, or the inside out. In other words, symptoms heal from a more important organ to a less important organ, and in the reverse order of their appearance in your body."

"I like what I hear, but I've gotta ask--if it's so effective, how can it not be just as dangerous?"

"Well, for example, traditional Western medicine works to eliminate a cancerous tumor through such invasive procedures as surgery, chemotherapy or radiation; homeopathy, on the other hand, gently re-oxygenates and stimulates the body's cells so its natural defenses cure the underlying state of 'dis-ease' that originally allowed the tumor to flourish."

"Because cancer cannot live in the presence of oxygen, right?"

"Right. Homeopathy has been proven effective over the centuries, and is relatively inexpensive. You can buy many common, every-day remedies without a prescription at your...."

"Local health-food store," Tom intoned.

"Right again," the doctor chuckled, "or at a homeopathic pharmacy. AIDS or cancer--or heart conditions-- should be treated by a qualified homeopathic physician, however, not by a self-guided hit-or-miss system, a health-food-store clerk--or even a medical doctor who has dabbled in homeopathy. Most M.D.s aren't sufficiently well-versed in the workings of constitutional problems, and could, consequently, be completely ineffective in recommending treatment. For serious illness, I'd recommend you look for a qualified homeopathic physician who has spent years beyond regular medical school in a homeopathic university. This person knows how to base treatment on the total person, not just the symptoms of the so-called 'disease.'"

"So, with that build-up, I take it you're going to give me the name of a real homeopathic doctor to see?"

Dr. Feelgood smiled. "How did you know? I can make certain recommendations, but I suggest that you see Dr. Soosamen. I think he's one of the best in this area. I've taken several classes in homeopathy, but, I repeat, with your kind of illness I think we should seek the advice of a medical doctor who has spent years of intensive study in a homeopathic university after finishing medical school, and who would know how to treat you properly."

"Doc, I appreciate your honesty."

"Tom, I appreciate your attitude."

20 - A KEY ELEMENT IN HEALING

"You know, doc, it's funny you should say that about my attitude, because I've always had a sign up on the wall of my office: IT'S ALL ATTITUDE."

"You're right--at least partially. Attitude--that is, a good attitude--is vital. While laughter can increase your sense of well-being, and even physically raise your immune system, hopelessness and depression have been scientifically proven to lower the body's immunity to disease. Did you know that?"

"Hey, I believe it."

"Attitude alone isn't enough, of course, but along with adequate rest and mild exercise, positive thinking can increase the activity of immune cells. But it works just as strong in reverse. A person can do all the right things--eat all the proper foods, take the necessary supplements, exercise regularly--yet still be unhealthy, or never heal properly from a dis-ease because his or her attitude is desperate and gloomy. When we think of and expect the worst, we set our bodies up for disease--and that is just what we get. So think positive thoughts!"

"Always! Except, of course, when I'm facing a knife. But I absolutely believe I can be healed, and I fully plan to be the master of my own destiny from here on out. What else can I do to make a quick recovery and rebuild this flabby body, besides the right attitude, proper exercise and real nutrition for my body?"

"Hey, that's a great start. If you begin thinking, right now, not about what you can put into your body, but what you can get out of it, you'll be on the healing path. Re-align your thoughts about food to realize that you must eat to live, not live to eat."

"How original."

"Hey, don't knock it if it works!"

21 - ANTIOXIDANTS

Tom dragged his feet over the threshold into Dr. Feelgood's office. "I barely made it here today, doc. I've got a horrible cold and I feel miserable. This kind of healing isn't working for me."

"Hey, back up a minute, Tom."

"No, you back up. You tell me to juice fruits and vegetables to clean the gunk out of my system, so I pull the juicer out of the closet, and I juice for the last three days. You tell me not to eat cheese, since it causes mucus to build up in my body, so I haven't been eating cheese for a couple of weeks. And I haven't had real ice cream--or milk. I've been good, really I have. So why is my whole body putting out so much mucus?" Tom sneezed violently.

"I shouldn't be going through this if I'm doing everything right," he yelled at the doctor. "Your medicine is worthless!"

"Are you finished, Tom?" Dr. Feelgood asked quietly.

"For now," Tom pouted.

"Good. Then let me tell you how happy I am that you're experiencing this so-called 'cold.'"

"You're happy? You're sick! No, I'm sick because you're sick! I don't know what I'm even saying, my head hurts so much. If I'm not blowing my nose, sneezing or coughing out crud, then I'm dealing with diarrhea. I'm sure it's because of this stupid juicing you're making me do."

"Hold on, Tom, I'm not making you do anything...."

"Oh, here we go again...it's my choice. All right, so my choosing to juice made me run to the bathroom last night for Imodium® more than once. It still didn't plug me up, though. That juice just doesn't like me--and I don't like the effect of it."

"Tom, please listen for a minute. I know you feel miserable because you're experiencing a 'cold.' Do you know how many billions of dollars have been spent on research to cure the common cold, and how unsuccessful this research has been?"

"No, and right now, I really don't care."

Dr. Feelgood smiled and went on. "The reason research has been unsuccessful in finding a cure for the common cold is because colds are actually cleansings. When a body becomes too toxic, or too plugged up by all the bad foods put into it, it goes through it's own elimination process. We call this elimination process a cold, because it has all the same symptoms--runny nose, itchy and weepy eyes, achy body from the possible fever associated with the cleansing."

"I'm sure I have a fever right now. I ache."

"I imagine you do. The fever is a result of the body's attempt to burn out the toxins invading it. It may be uncomfortable, but it is a wonderful tool created by the human body to clean itself up and return it to better shape. Once again you fell back into your old habits last night and ran to your medicine cabinet to suppress something your body needed to do, and was doing naturally."

"Well, my body's not making me very happy right now."

"So sorry, dear Tom. The juicing you're blaming for your diarrhea is most likely loosening things up in your intestines that have been sitting there for a long time, and cleaning them out. A very good sign, as far as I'm concerned. The toxins are being flushed out, which is exactly what we want. Just make sure you continue replacing the fluids you're losing with the diarrhea. If you always get it when you juice, back off a little bit. Put a little less of the beet in with the carrot, for instance--whatever it takes. Remember, I said you'd have to continually experiment to see what's best for your body."

Tom sneezed so hard he rocked in his chair, then blew his nose. He shook his head in amazement. "So, a cold is a good thing?"

"Usually. Of course, some colds are associated with viral pneumonia, and have to be treated differently. In general, though, take care of your cold with extra rest, vitamins, and lots of fluids, such as fresh-pressed juices, herb teas, and lots of water, maybe with a little lemon squeezed into it. As a matter of fact, I'd like to see you do some Vitamin C Therapy."

"Which means...?"

"T-helper cells, along with B-cells and macrophages, are white-blood cells (leukocytes). They help protect your body against invading bacteria and viruses. Large doses of Vitamin C--as massive as your bowel will tolerate--can aid in T-helper-cell stabilization. The sicker a person, the more Vitamin C is needed to fight off infection."

"At least this stuff isn't new, Doc. Everybody knows you take Vitamin C when you get a cold or the flu, which I've been doing."

"That's good, and you're right, but it's not only

for air-borne viruses. Vitamin C is a natural antioxidant, which helps fight all anaerobic infections."

"Isn't too much vitamin C dangerous?"

"Yes and no."

Tom groaned. "Not again!"

"When your tissues are sufficiently saturated with vitamin C, you might experience diarrhea, which, if too extensive, can cause dehydration. That can be dangerous if you don't rehydrate with extra fluids. The runs will stop, though, when your gastrointestinal tract has used up the vitamin C fighting the disease. Tests have shown that a healthy person who tolerates Vitamin C can take 10 to 20 grams without getting diarrhea. A person with a mild cold can take 30 to 60 grams in 24 hours with no side effects; someone with a severe cold, 100 grams; a person with influenza, 150 grams; and patients with mononucleosis or viral pneumonia can take up to or even over 200 grams in 24 hours--that's almost half a pound."

"The sicker you are, the more you can take?"

"Right. Your increased tolerance to the vitamin indicates how it's being used as a free-radical scavenger during these toxic conditions. Two grams of Vitamin C every hour won't cure a severe cold, but

60 to 70 grams every 24 hours will."

"Just what is a free-radical scavenger?"

"Good question. First, let me explain what a free radical is."

"Good idea."

"A free radical is any molecule with an oxygen atom that's missing an electron. The oxygen atom goes crazy trying to replace the missing electron. The only place it can find one is in a healthy molecule. In other words, free radicals are free-roaming molecules that, if unchecked, can damage cells, produce genetic changes, and even cause cancer. Illness, injury, surgery, and even some allergic reactions produce free radicals, which burn up the body's Vitamin C, and, in turn, cause more dis-ease. Free radicals basically are, in fact, the underlying cause of all diseases. Our bodies are full of them--we all have billions of free radicals attacking our healthy cells all the time. Antioxidants are one of the quickest ways to disarm them, and vitamin C is one of the most powerful antioxidants you can take. Many AIDS patients become allergic to their antibiotics, because they take them when they're very sick. Massive doses of vitamin C, which scavenge free radicals, can disarm these unwanted antibodies, and, at the same time, step up the immune system's attack on the parasite."

"Is that all? I just need vitamin C?"

"Plus up to 83,000 units per day of beta-carotene (which converts to vitamin A); as well as at least 400 mg. of vitamin E. I'd also like to see you take 200 mcg. of selenium and 100 mg. of zinc every day. You should add those to any supplement list. They all stimulate the immune system and promote microbial activity against viruses or parasites; they're all antioxidants. You don't have to take them only in supplement capsule form, though. You can also get them in everyday foods.

- **Vitamin A**
    Cayenne, Dandelion, Eyebright, Grape Leaves, Okra Pods, Paprika, Parsley, Red Raspberry.

Vitamin A is destroyed by alcohol, coffee, cortisone and Vitamin D deficiency.

- **Vitamin C**
    Elderberries, Rose Hips, Watercress.

Vitamin C is destroyed by tobacco, antibiotics, aspirin and cortisone.

- **Vitamin D**
    Alfalfa, Lettuce, Sunshine or Sunlight.

- **Vitamin E**
    Red Raspberry, Rose Hips.

You can destroy both Vitamin D & E by taking mineral oil.

"I had no idea alcohol, caffeine, mineral oil, tobacco and cortisone could destroy the effectiveness of vitamins! I haven't been doing much right in the past, I'm coming to realize."

"But you're learning now, so you won't have any excuse in the future. So, do you think you understand what free radicals are now?"

"Sure. Free radicals are the bad guys--bad cells--that cause destruction in the body. To disarm them, you've gotta take the good guys--the scavengers that eat up the free radicals. And the scavengers are antioxidants, like vitamins C, A and E, beta-carotene, selenium and zinc. Right?"

"Right. Very good. How about a lunch break? I'll see you here in, say, an hour and a half."

"Sounds good. In the meantime, I'm off to the

health-food store--to pick up some antioxidants!"

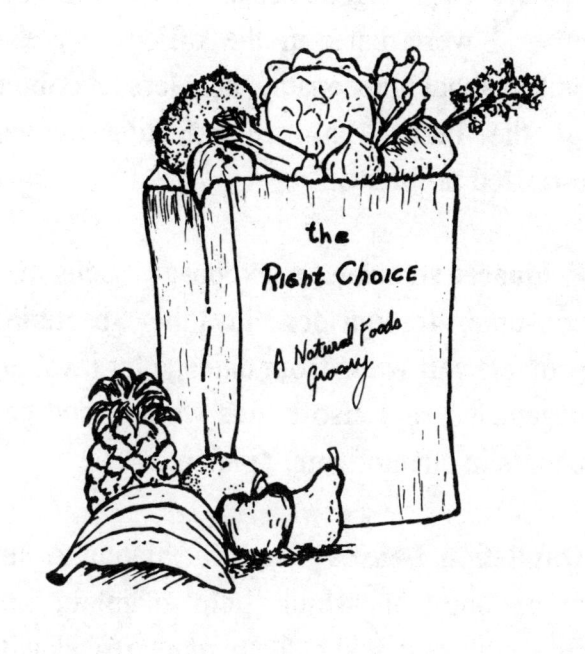

22 - HERBS & MUSHROOMS

"Natural healing offers a lot of choices," Dr. Feelgood began once he and Tom were back in the office. "We've already talked about homeopathy; now let's talk about some of the herbs that are effective against immune-related problems:

- **Echinacea** stimulates macrophages (cells that consume foreign or invading bacteria), protects cell walls from damage by invading organisms, and also builds white blood cell counts in chemotherapy patients.

- **Dandelion Leaves** - high in vitamin A and zinc, both of which help maintain cell integrity, and make them more resistant to invasion or breakdown.

- **Siberian Ginseng** works indirectly on the immune system by toning the hormonal system that, in turn, helps the body adapt to stress.

- **Lomatium**, a native American herb, can inactivate viruses--a property found in few herbs or conventional drugs. It contains oils with carbon-ring chemical structures that interfere with virus growth, without damaging normal tissue.

- **Pau D'Arco**, which can be made into a fine-tasting tea, is not only rich in oxygen, but also in a class of chemicals known as quinones, which can destroy certain fungi and bacteria.

- **Goldenseal**, one of the most bitter herbs, is a powerful tonic, or herbal antibiotic. It kills microbes, strengthens the body's ability to fight infection, activates the white blood cells, and reduces fever.

- **Astragalus** works to strengthen the immune system on a deep level, rebuilding the bone-marrow reserve.

- **Burdock Root** acts on the same level as astragalus, and is a powerful blood cleanser as well.

- **Garlic** is one of nature's blood cleansers and purifiers, potent and powerful. Commonly used to tone the heart and build up the immune system, it improves T-cells and candidia conditions, reduces fever, and acts as an antibiotic, anti-microbial, and anti-viral agent in man. It can help diminish much of the acute pathology associated with the devastating family of viruses closely allied with HIV infection. Garlic contains therapeutic factors of germanium, magnesium and selenium as well as 17 amino acids, 33 sulfur compounds and vitamins B1, A and C.

- **Cayenne** (red pepper) is one of the most healing agents known to man--and one of the most misunderstood. A synergistic herb, cayenne increases the effectiveness of other herbs in the body. Cayenne is also the greatest heart strengthener found in most spice cabinets. Anyone with an ailing heart can rapidly strengthen it by taking cayenne on a consistent basis. Cayenne has stopped heart attacks, and deep-wound bleeding without burning the wound site. Fine restaurants often keep it in the kitchen as a first-aid treatment for employees who injure themselves with knives and other sharp instruments.

"Geez, that's quite a list," Tom said in astonishment.

"That's barely touching the surface, Tom."

"I didn't realize there were so many natural ways to heal--although I should have, I guess. After all, people have been using herbs since earliest times. All those legends about the ayurvedic medicines being thousands of years old, and shamans going out and looking for different plant leaves and roots were for real, huh?"

"Absolutely. And while herbs alone can't cure everything, they are just as effective as drugs--if not more so--and ordinarily have no side-effects at all. Of course, they can be also be abused like drugs, if not taken in proper dosages. They're not to be taken lightly, because they are very potent."

"So they're just like taking safe drugs, right?"

"Oh, no. Herbs don't act in the same way as conventional drugs. Many different constituents of an herb interact to work against complex diseases. They are considerably milder than drugs--they never overpower the body, or drain its energy. We call them 'alteratives,' and that's what they really are. You take them over a period of time, and they gradually alter the body's functioning. They are not a 'quick fix'--and they won't work well if you are trashing your body in other ways at the same time."

"Okay, doc, I've already gotten that point. I'm eating much better, and I'm doing the juicing, even though it's making me sick--and it tastes worse than I expected."

"Yes, raw juice is sometimes an acquired taste--although many love it from the first time they drink it--but it's worth the effort. Herbs are normally taken in tablets, capsules or liquid extract preserved in organic alcohol, so you don't have to worry about how your palate responds."

"I suppose you're going to tell me the ones you want me to take, and how much of each?"

"Absolutely. I'll give you a specific list before you leave today. But the herbs I mentioned as being immune stimulants are just a few of those that can help rebuild your immune system. Several types of mushrooms are as good as herbs for treating serious conditions."

"Don't mushrooms give you hallucinations?"

"Certainly not all types! You eat mushrooms on your salads, don't you, or on your pizza?"

"Oh, yeah, that's right."

"There are varieties that cause hallucinations, but I'm not talking about those, or about the standard button mushrooms you usually cut up for salads. I'm talking about Shiitake and Ganaderma mushrooms, both of which are very important in treating cancer and AIDS because of their anti-viral and anti-cancer properties. You can find extracts from the shiitake mushroom, called L.E.M., in health-food stores. In fact, another product designed to boost the immune system is a combination of five different mushrooms: ganaderma, shiitake, polyporus, tremella and poria, although I don't remember its exact name. You can find that at your health-food store, too. If you want, you can even look for these in their fresh, natural state and add them to your diet. Many supermarkets carry at least shiitake mushrooms now as a matter of course. They taste good, and you get their healing benefits on top of it."

"Don't you remember, you said I should rotate those mushrooms around in my diet? Well, I've been eating them. They're one of the few things about this whole thing that I actually enjoy. In fact, I love them."

"Good. Bon Appetit!"

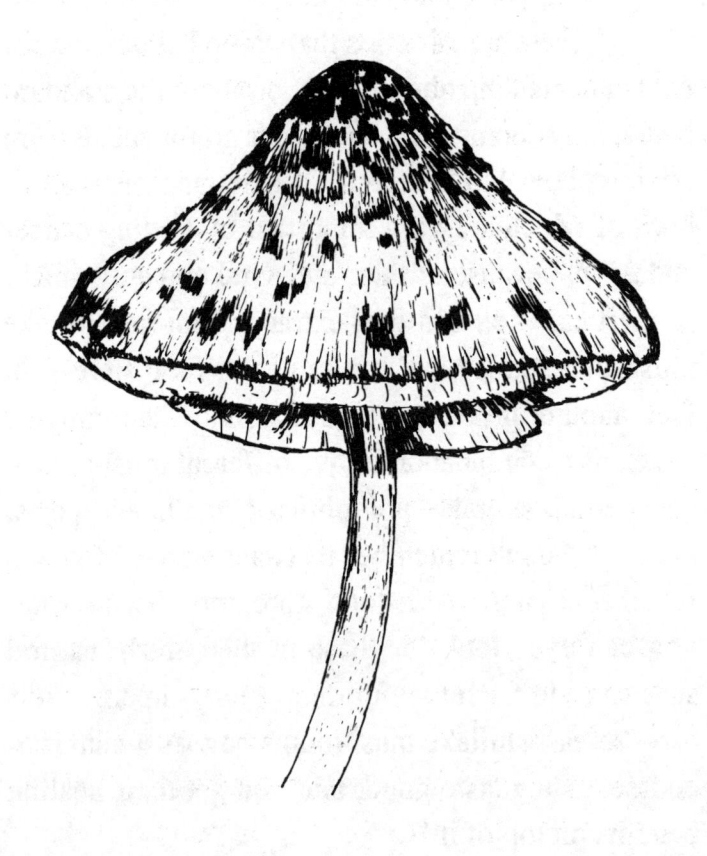

23 - HYDROGEN PEROXIDE

Tom sat back in his chair, looking rather satisfied. "So," he said, "I give up smoking permanently--which I'm committed to, doc. I haven't had one in three days now--and give up all my lovely high-fat foods, and drink more filtered water, and eat the right food, and get the right amount of exercise, and take the herbs you give me on the list, and drink the fresh fruit and vegetable juices, and take my antioxidants and see a homeopath--this is quite a program, even without the enemas or colonics. That pretty much wraps it up, right?"

"Well, yes and no."

Tom groaned. "I shoulda known!"

"First, let me congratulate you on quitting smoking. I knew you had what it takes to quit--the will power and control--keep it up! Now, did you know, Tom," Dr. Feelgood went on with a smile, "that our bodies are composed mostly of water?"

"Yeah, we're ugly bags of mostly water--I got

that from a Star Trek episode."

"And did you know that water that is constantly rushing, such as rain, snow and mountain streams, contains natural hydrogen peroxide?"

"Hydrogen peroxide? The stuff you use to clean cuts and dye hair?"

"Exactly. The water's rapid agitation forms the hydrogen peroxide (H_2O_2), which then kills any harmful microbes present. That's why the water from mountain streams always tastes so good. Now, of all the elements the body needs, only oxygen is in such constant demand that its absence brings death in minutes. For the human body to become a medium for parasites, the oxygen-saturation level of its fluids has to drop well below the optimum level for healthy cell growth and function."

"And since cancer is anaerobic, that's when it would grow, right? When the body's oxygen level is way below normal?"

"Right."

"So, my oxygen level got really low, allowing the free radicals to take hold of my healthy cells, and that's why I got cancer."

"In a nutshell, yes. Now, have you ever heard of using hydrogen peroxide to restore the oxygen balance back to normal?"

"Like I said, I've only heard about using it to clean a cut, or dye your hair. Oh, I've also heard it's very toxic if you drink it."

"Very true. When concentrated, H_2O_2 is highly toxic. When diluted to therapeutic levels, though, it's completely non-toxic, and uniquely beneficial. So, for example, if you put anywhere from one to eight pints of 3% H_2O_2 (which is what you commonly find in your grocery/drugstore) in a bathtub half full of water, you could soak in it, and absorb the oxygen."

"Through your skin?"

"Why not? The skin is the body's largest organ, after all."

"I knew that. So why didn't I think of that?"

"You can also use H_2O_2 orally, too, which will boost your oxygen level and revitalize normal cells, while killing pathogens and viruses. If you do take it orally, though, you have to be prepared for a slight feeling of nausea while the H_2O_2 is liberating the free oxygen, especially if you have a high level of toxins, virus or streptococcus in your stomach."

"How do you know what kind to use?"

"Food grade H_2O_2 (35%) is better for internal use, but...you know, this stuff is very dangerous if not diluted properly. Rather than lay out exactly how to do it, I'd rather you just realize that H_2O_2 therapy is very effective for increasing oxygen levels high enough that free radicals are actually eliminated from the body."

"That's pretty powerful stuff! I'd almost be afraid to try it."

"Yes, it is powerful, and no, I don't want you doing hydrogen-peroxide therapy at this point. It's nothing to mess around with if you don't have the proper supervision, and right now I think you've got enough to tackle with the diet changes, juicing and antioxidants. I just wanted you to know that there's always more you can do to help clean, rebuild and maintain your body's health. Never think you've learned it all."

"Hey, doc, I wasn't serious. I mean, I can see there's so much more to know. I've got the feeling I'm going to be reading and talking to people and studying for the rest of my life!"

"And if you stay on this course, it'll be a nice, long life."

"Amen to that, doc, amen to that."

24 - ARTHRITIS

"Listen, Tom, we're just about at the point where we can stop the marathon sessions, and get down to a more reasonable meeting schedule. Besides that, I think it's just about time for you to get back to work, although I hope you'll go back with a new attitude--less stressed and more energized."

"It couldn't be any other way at this point, could it?"

"Now, you know I've got a reference library here that you can tap into any time you want, Tom. There are also plenty of other sources you can go to: bookstores, natural-foods stores or health-food stores, libraries and especially friends who are in the know, such as Dana...or Carlene."

"I'll call Carlene when I get home, and see if I can browse through her library."

"Good. Knowing Carlene, she'll be willing to share and help you along. The more you know, the better you'll be able to be your own doctor most of the time, and not always be a victim--either of doctors who are victims of drug and insurance companies, or of advertising."

"You know, doc, I used to think school was just important for kids. But we all have to keep learning and educating ourselves just to survive. I thought I knew more when I was 16 than I do now at 45. Hey, before I go, I've got one more thing I'd like to talk to you about today."

"Shoot."

"I think I've got a little touch of arthritis in my shoulder. And maybe in my hands and knees. I don't really know. I've been taking prednisone for awhile, but at this point, I have to believe there's something better for me than taking a steriod--and stopping salt."

"Yes, there definitely is. You know, arthritis isn't as great a killer as cancer, AIDS or even heart disease, but it is perhaps the most crippling and agonizing of all degenerative dis-eases, causing more pain, despair and suffering than any other. Do you know what arthritis is?"

"Pain, swelling...pain. That pretty much lays it out for me. Pain."

"That pretty much lays it out for everyone. Swelling, pain, stiffness--arthritis is essentially a degenerative process that inflames the joints."

"Inflammation. That's me, all right. Especially first thing in the morning. I can even tell you when it's about to rain. Like this is something I want to be able to do!"

"Well, you know, it's not incurable."

"I had a feeling you were going to say that....I was hoping you were going to say that."

"As with most of the other dis-eases we've discussed, relief is usually sought for the symptoms, without looking into or eliminating the underlying cause or causes. Physicians and arthritis sufferers hailed the discovery of cortisone (similar to prednisone) as a long-sought miracle cure--just as they had previously hailed sulfa drugs, gold injections, and...."

"And copper bracelets."

"But of course, we don't want to forget copper bracelets. Eventually, though, all these so-called treatments have proven to be cruel disappointments, as you no doubt already know. Not one of them offers permanent relief. Cortisone, in fact, soon proved to be a worse remedy than the dis-ease, with all its toxic reactions and dangerous side-effects, and is considered on its way out in the treatment of arthritis, by the way."

"What's in?"

"Nothing across-the-board, as far as traditional medicine is concerned, but some arthritis sufferers are discovering that their condition is a systemic, metabolic dis-ease--the end result of longtime abuse of normal bodily processes. It's not going to be cured by a single miracle drug."

"So the same stuff I'm doing to heal the cancer and my heart..."

"Exactly. Correct and eliminate the underlying causes and abnormal conditions that brought on the arthritis, and you eliminate the actual condition."

"I get it. So arthritis is the same thing. I've messed up my body, and when I un-mess it, my joints will feel better along with all the rest."

"Well, I think I would have put it more scientifically, but that's the main idea, yes. Medicine-at-large is in the dark about the causes and effective treatments for arthritis, but naturopathic and biologically-oriented practitioners have developed simple, biologic methods of treatment that have proven to be most successful in treating and eliminating arthritis, along with many other dis-eases."

"Yeah, that's scientific enough."

Dr. Feelgood laughed. "The point is, for all of Western medicine's miraculous discoveries, drugs are not the wonders we once thought. Drugs will not heal dis-eases. Only when the body's own healing forces are assisted and supported can we achieve lasting results. Treatments have to be directed at correcting the underlying causes of the given disorder, and strengthening the patient's immune system with proper rest, exercise, and natural, whole, fresh foods, plus the proper supplements to support those foods."

"So, specifically for my arthritis..."

"Fresh-pressed fruit and vegetable juices are wonderful healers for arthritic pain, as they tend to wash away and dissolve encrusted calcium deposits, and thus eliminate the joint inflammation. It's merely a question of drinking enough. A small glass of concentrated orange juice won't do it."

"Don't worry, doc, I'm drinking my juices."

"Good. Try juicing some grapefruit. Even if you don't want to take the time to buy another citrus juicer and juice it yourself, you can always buy the fresh-squeezed grapefruit juice at your natural-foods store--just remember **not** to buy it canned, and remember to look at the date it was made so you buy it fresh. The organic salicylic acid in fresh grapefruit is especially good for dissolving the foreign-matter accumulation in joint cartilage."

"No problem. I've always liked grapefruit. And citrus juicers are reasonably priced, so I'll pick another one up. When I get back to work, if I don't have the time to make it at home, maybe I can send one of my gofers to the store for some while I'm walking laps around the lot," Tom grinned.

"Good. I think you'll find that if you keep on this program, you won't be able to predict the weather so well in a few weeks."

"Aw, gee, what a shame!"

"You know, Tom, as you progress along this path, people are going to start asking what you're doing, or what 'miracle drug' you're taking. They'll notice your increased energy, your better coloring...."

"Yeah, some of my friends are already telling me I don't look so pasty, so I guess the oxygen must be reaching some of my body's cells....I never knew I looked pasty...."

"See how quickly natural healing can bring you back to life? There's nothing wrong with spreading the word--although a lot of people will doubt you or think you're crazy."

"Hey, doc, I'm going to tell them the whole story: how I'm eating, what I'm not eating anymore, the juices, the exercise, the thing about the water, the antioxidants, the herbs, the homeopathy, the whole works. And if I can get them even a little bit interested, I'm gonna bring them here to meet you. But most of all, I'm going to do my best to convince them that I had a choice--and they have a choice. After all, that's what life is really all about, isn't it? We all have a choice!"

"Amen to that, my friend. Amen to that."

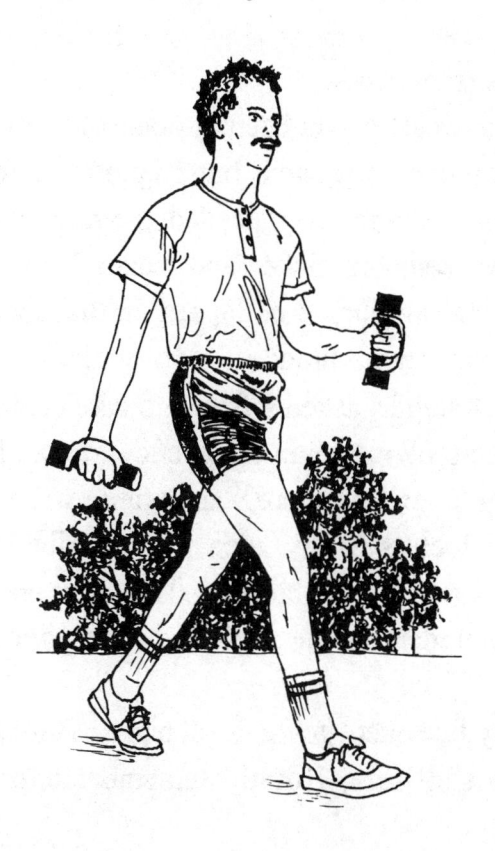

CHOICES WE MADE (Author & Editor)

B*era's Story* . . . I was 24 years old, invincible and tireless. I thought I could keep going 24 hours a day and never go down.

I was wrong.

The weather had been atrocious for 3 weeks. My lungs were congested, but I couldn't afford to miss work--I desperately needed the money. The more I worked, the sicker and sicker I got. One evening, still at work, I collapsed on the floor, and started coughing up blood. So dizzy that I couldn't stand up straight, I asked a friend to take me home--instead, he took me to an emergency room. The x-ray of my lungs said there was nothing wrong with me. The doctors had no idea why my ribs hurt so much, or why I couldn't breathe. They sent me home with a reminder to take aspirin for the pain in my ribs.

My fever kept going up all night. Through my dizziness and haze, I dimly remember telling my mother that I didn't feel very good and couldn't breathe very well. She called a homeopathic doctor, who made a housecall to see me. Checking my lungs and the x-rays I had brought home from the hospital, he advised me that, in addition to a 105^0 fever, I had double pneumonia, intercostal neuralgia and pleurisy. As he left, he cautioned me to not leave my house again until I was well--as if I could have walked out the door on my own! The doctor came over every morning for 9 days straight, and as my healing progressed, new homeopathic remedies were administered. I can still remember the constant, excruciating pain, and not being able to get a deep, cleansing or satisfying breath. All I knew was that I wanted to die to escape the pain. My mother slept on my floor for 11 nights, expecting me to expire at any moment. I lost 14 pounds off an already thin frame, dropping down to 96 lbs. at 5'6". I've burned all the pictures taken of me during that time--I looked like I was from Auschwitz.

Had it not been for Dr. Smith, my homeopathic doctor who retired soon thereafter, I don't think I would have lived to write this book.

For obvious reasons, my interest in natural methods of healing was born during that time. Fascinated--and thankful--I simply had to know more. I went back to school, and eventually obtained my degree in naturopathy. But before I was graduated, I was presented with another opportunity from which to learn.

It was a day like any other February day, except that I couldn't get out of bed. The pain in my back was excruciating and incapacitating. I had no idea what I had done to cause such pain in my lower back. I called my fiance to let him know I was in real trouble--I couldn't move! Rushing over, he found me still in bed, unable to move, and unable to be moved without screaming in agony.

We went to an orthopedic specialist first, but he could not find anything wrong on the x-rays of my back. We went to acupuncturists, followed by chiropractors--anyone who might have an answer. The wedding was in two months, and I wanted to be able to walk down the aisle, but since no one could come up with an answer to my pain, I figured I must be dying of some horrible disease--much worse than cancer, I was sure--that was eating up my back. I told my fiance I couldn't marry him with this problem. He wanted to get married anyway. He believed we'd find an answer.

I lived, went to school and worked in constant pain for the next four months. I could barely move.

I wanted to die from the neverending pain. Finally, a natural healer, a gentleman well into his 70s who was about to perform acupuncture on my back, realized that my problem was not in my back at all. He proved his theory by touching a spot on the calf of my right leg that actually increased the pain, and explained that this was the meridian where my nerve circuitry to the female organs was located--he had felt the heat emanating from the right side of my abdomen. He immediately advised me to go to my gynecologist, which I did.

The first gynecologist I visited said I had a cyst on my right ovary that was as large as my fist, and that required immediate surgery. I went for a second opinion--and got the same answer. In fact, the 3rd, 4th and 5th doctors each said something worse than the last, finally concluding with the "fact" that I needed a hysterectomy. I had another opinion-- that I might want a family.

Depressed, I went back to the man who had originally discovered the nature of my pain. He said acupuncture would help somewhat, but to speed things along, I should seek the treatment of a qualified homeopathist. But my homeopathist had retired! Fortunately, my mother had just made the acquaintance of a new homeopathist, and was very happy with her. Thank God! This homeopathic doctor immediately put me on a remedy that started shrinking the cyst. Each day I felt a little less pressure. Three weeks later, the only pain I had left was from the scar tissue left by the cyst. My homeopathist had also figured out that I had a pretty severe case of endometriosis, and wanted to work on eliminating that problem, too. She did.

I never took a drug. I never had a hysterectomy. I never had any surgery. I only took homeopathic remedies. Today I have no signs of endometriosis remaining, nor have I had another sign of any more cyst formations. My husband and I have celebrated our tenth wedding anniversary feeling healthfully vibrant and alive.

I could go on and on about my health experiences, but I would like you to hear from my editor. Not only is Claudia Suzanne a very talented writer and editor, but she is a living example of the power of natural healing in her own life. I already loved her work, much of which I had read, and because of her proud, loving spirit, and what she has overcome in her own health, I simply had to have her as my editor for *I Have A Choice?!* Read on and see why.

Bera Dordoni

Claudia's Story... The last time I saw a doctor was when some neurologist at Cigna Health told me to reconcile myself to a wheelchair. That was over five years ago. You see, I have multiple sclerosis, a degenerative disease that could, indeed, have put me into a wheelchair some time ago. At the very least, I should be having balance problems, and requiring the occasional use of a cane or walker. I should also, by now, be having consistent bladder-control problems, and have lost the vision in my one weak eye. I should be fighting constant fatigue, and should experience a significant increase in my MS symptoms following any bout with a cold or the flu. Since I also have thoracic outlet compression, I should be in pretty much constant pain whenever I tax my right arm, and with my tachycardia, I should have chest pains and a rapid pulse whenever I exert myself or get stressed out. To top it off, with my diagnosis of Reynaud's Disease, I should be unable to function during winter, and should be constantly on the lookout for signs of Lupus. In other words, I should be a total physical--not to mention emotional and mental--mess.

I have none of the above. I repeat, *none* of the above. I have had them all--and more--but after a great deal of reading, trial and error, and work with my naturopath to find the right combination of supplements and proper foods--which, by the way, needs to be reworked and modified from time to time--I now enjoy extremely good health, vibrant energy, and no--N-O, NO--apparent degeneration from any of my dis-eases. No, during my initial recovery, I did not eat meat. Yes, now, during my maintenance, I do--in fact, as an MS patient, I have found it is vital for me to eat liver and shellfish on a regular basis. Every dis-ease is different. So is every body.

Some MS patients have one attack, and never have another problem for the rest of their lives. I am not one of those people, and, in fact, still have to cope with what I now call my "physical inconveniences" every day. For instance, extreme heat wears me out almost immediately. Extreme cold will trigger a Reynaud's attack--and extreme cold for me is not as extreme as for the average person. The difference is that with my hard-won knowledge of healing, I now know how to counteract those attacks, and can regain my equilibrium quickly, with no ill after-effects--a remarkable feat I certainly could not claim as true five years ago. I must keep up with my regimen, or my inconveniences will get the better of me--and I've fallen off the wagon enough times to have proven it. However, I've also recovered from those falls remarkably quickly, because I have built up my body's strength and immune system so well, even I would have a hard time doing myself in at this point.

Five years ago, I was faced with nothing but pain, despair, poverty-inducing medical expenses, and hopelessness. The choices given to me by my half-dozen "traditional" doctors were pain-killers, steroids, appliances and experimental drugs. Today I lead an active, fulfilling life that is dependent on such "voo-doo" tactics as healthy foods, herbal supplements, homeopathic remedies, moderation of my "evil" vices (sugar and extra beef), exercise and a happy, positive attitude. I have built a career from the ground up, am raising a family, and enjoy a varied and productive social life.

I made the choice to take control of my life.
You can, too.

Claudia Suzanne

KEYS TO A HEALTHY LIFE

Carrot juice

The number one blood cleanser in the vegetable kingdom, carrot juice is almost chemically identical to our blood's hemoglobin, so it is easily recognized by the body's cells. Carrot juice quickly breaks down and eliminates mucus from the body.

Exercise daily

If you cannot do vigorous exercise, take a good walk. Exercise gets the oxygen moving in the body, washes out toxins, and builds and strengthens bones and muscles.

Oxygenate the Body

Avoid foods devoid of live enzymes. Smoking and drinking alcohol block oxygen--so does eating "dead" foods, which have been cooked so much they do not have any live enzymes left.

Believe in Your Healing Method

Have the right attitude toward your method of treatment, and believe in it wholly, or it will not be as effective. Look at illness by thinking of the body as being out of balance--out of ease...not at ease...in a state of dis-ease. The situation will not feel so threatening and overpowering to the point where you'll accept a "death sentence" at face value. Get to work putting your body back in balance.

Symptoms are Warning Signs

Deal with the underlying cause of the dis-ease. Drugs merely mask symptoms, which does not aid in actual recovery. Drugs, in fact, can destroy the body's own natural defenses, and weaken the immune system. Eliminate the cause of the disorder, and the symptoms will disappear.

Liquid Nourishment

Wheatgrass juice is a wonderful blood cleanser. Even closer chemically to the blood's hemoglobin than carrot juice, it is the most natural destroyer of cancer and other blood maladies that exists.

Antioxidants

Having the ability to halt the destruction of free radicals in the body, vitamins A, C and E, and beta-carotene, selenium and zinc should be taken daily.

Avoid Tap Water At All Costs

The lead and chlorine in most municipal water supplies are carcinogens the body can live without.

Food Substitutes

Substitutes for allergy-causing foods are readily available, and quite enjoyable to eat and drink.

Proper Food Combining

Eating in the right combinations can give a person more energy than he or she ever thought possible, while aiding digestion and contributing to a general feeling of well-being.

Whatever the source of your discomfort, remember this:

You are a Total Person, NOT a Disease. When the Total Person is Treated, the Odds Are in That Person's Favor For Recovery. Above All, Stop Buying the Idea that Cancer, AIDS and Other "Terminal" Illnesses are Automatic Death Sentences!!!

REFERENCES

Airola, Paavo, N.D. *How to Get Well*. Heath Plus Publishers, Oregon, 1974.

Airola, Paavo, N.D. *There Is A Cure For Arthritis*. Parker Publishing, New York, 1968.

Berger, Stuart M., M.D. *How to Be Your Own Nutritionist*. Avon Books, New York, 1987.

Berger, Stuart M., M.D. *Dr. Berger's Immune Power Diet*. Signet Books, New York, 1986.

Bieler, Henry G., M.D. *Food is Your Best Medicine*. Ballantine Books, New York, 1983.

Christopher, Dr. John R. *Secrets of a Master Herbalist*. Christopher Publications, Utah, 1983.

Diamond, Harvey and Marilyn. *Fit For Life*. Warner Books, New York, 1987.

Gerson, Max, M.D., *A Cancer Therapy*. Gerson Institute, California, 1st Ed 1958, 2nd Ed 1990.

Greer, Joseph H., M.D. *A Physician In The House*. U.S.A. Publishers, 1940.

Hamlyn, Edward C., M.D. *The Healing Art of Homeopathy*. Keats Publishing, Connecticut.

Kushi, Michio. *The Macrobiotic Way*. Avery Publishing Group Inc., New York, 1985, 1993.

Leichtberg, J., M.D. *How to Los Weight Healthfully Without Dieting*. Medicus Formulas, Inc. and J. Leichtberg, M.D., California, 1993.

Mae, Eydie with Loeffler, Chris. *How I Conquered Cancer Naturally*. Harvest House Publishers, Oregon, 1975.

Mendelsohn, Robert S., M.D. *Confessions of a Medical Heretic.* Warner Books, New York, 1979.

Quinn, Dick. *Left for Dead.* R.F. Quinn Publishing Co., Minnesota, 1992.

Sattilaro, Anthony J., M.D. *Recalled by Life.* Avon Books, New York, 1982.

Shadman, Alonzo J., M.D. *Who Is Your Doctor and Why?* Pivot Health Editions, Connecticut, 1980.

Siegel, Bernie S., M.D. *Love, Medicine & Miracles.* Harper & Row, Publishers, New York, 1986.

Vogel, Dr. H.C.A.. *The Nature Doctor, A Manual of Traditional and Complementary Medicine.* Keats Publishing, Inc., Connecticut, 1952, 1991.

Vithoulkas, George, M.I.H. *Homeopathy: Medine of the New Man.* Arco Publishing, Inc., New York, 1979.

Walker, Dr. Norman W., D.Sc., R.D. Pope, M.D. *Fresh Vegetable and Fruit Juices.* Norwalk Press, Arizona, 1978.

Whitaker, Julian, M.D. *Health and Healing - Tomorrow's Medicine Today* Newsletters

Willix, Jr., Robert D., M.D. *You Can Feel Good All The Time.* Dr. Willix's Health For Life LLC, Maryland, 1994.

The Beron Foundation ... Working to bring you a choice.

The promotion of balance and harmony between man and his environment is necessary for the recovery of those whose lives are being lived in a state of dis-ease and stress. We at The Beron Foundation and B.F. Publishing firmly believe that education is the key to preventing dis-ease and dis-harmony, and are here to provide a network for those in need of vital information regarding all the choices one has when it comes to one's own personal health care. Concentration is made in the areas of 'alternative' approaches to achieving maximum health.

One of the fundamental premises of the Beron Foundation's teachings is the idea that each person might consider taking at least partial responsibility for his or her state of dis-ease or dis-ability and the recovery therefrom.

For more information from the Beron Foundation in the areas of natural alternative approaches to healing including nutrition, preventative-health maintenance, weight-loss management, and attitude and lifestyle adjustment for the total person, please contact the Foundation's toll-free line (800) 544-7264 or write to us at P.O. Box 2712-344, Huntington Beach, California 92647.

The Beron Foundation thanks the donors who recognize that we are a non-profit foundation working to bring you a choice.

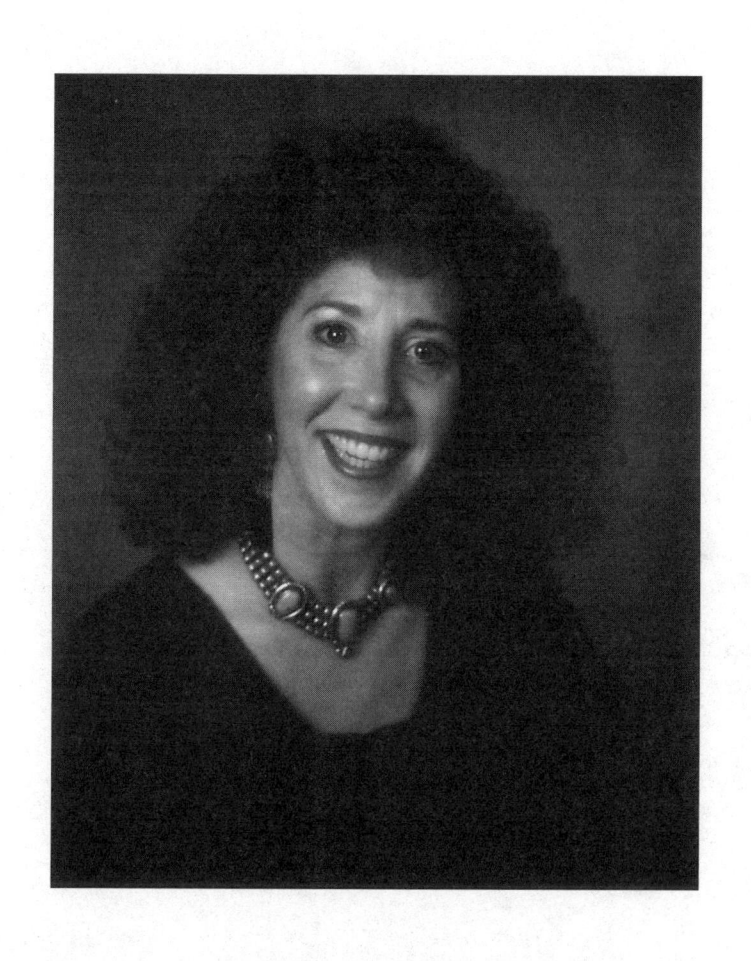

It's your choice now!

Bera

I Have a Choice?!

Order form to share with your friends.

☐ **YES,** rush my order for ____ copy(ies) of *I Have A Choice?!*
☐ to me, or ☐ send as a gift to a friend.

Book $12.95 ea. $_____

☐ **YES,** I want to take advantage of the new subscription rate for your newsletter informing me about new and alternative approaches to healing. I understand that if I am not completely satisfied, I can get a full refund within the first 90 days of my subscription.

One-Year Subscription $15.00 $_____

☐ **YES,** I firmly believe that education is the key to preventing dis-ease and dis-harmony, and that when the body is in balance, it is healthy. I want to help continue your commitment to disseminate educational information, create public awareness in the area of natural healing and promote research to find new and alternative approaches to healing.

Enclosed is my pledge of $_____

Add $4.00 S&H per book order $_____

CA residence add 7.75% sales tax $_____

TOTAL AMOUNT DUE $_____

Name_____

Street Address_____
(No P.O. Box Address)

City _____ State _____ Zip _____

Daytime Phone ( ) _____
(In case we have a question about your order.)

Payment Method:

☐ Check or money order payable to B.F. Publishing.
☐ Charge my ☐ MasterCard ☐ VISA ☐ Amex

Card # _____ Exp. Date_____

Signature_____

SEND ORDER TO: B.F. Publishing
P.O. Box 2712-344
Huntington Beach, CA 92647
800-544-7264

I Have a Choice?!
Order form to share with your friends.

☐ **YES,** rush my order for ____ copy(ies) of *I Have A Choice?!*
  ☐ to me, or ☐ send as a gift to a friend.
                                    Book $12.95 ea. $_____

☐ **YES,** I want to take advantage of the new subscription rate for your newsletter informing me about new and alternative approaches to healing. I understand that if I am not completely satisfied, I can get a full refund within the first 90 days of my subscription.
                        One-Year Subscription $15.00 $_____

☐ **YES,** I firmly believe that education is the key to preventing dis-ease and dis-harmony, and that when the body is in balance, it is healthy. I want to help continue your commitment to disseminate educational information, create public awareness in the area of natural healing and promote research to find new and alternative approaches to healing.
                            Enclosed is my pledge of $_____

                    Add $4.00 S&H per book order $_____

                    CA residence add 7.75% sales tax $_____

                            TOTAL AMOUNT DUE $_____

Name_____

Street Address_____
           (No P.O. Box Address)
City _____ State _____ Zip _____

Daytime Phone ( ) _____
              (In case we have a question about your order.)
Payment Method:
☐ Check or money order payable to B.F. Publishing.
☐ Charge my ☐ MasterCard ☐ VISA ☐ Amex

Card # _____ Exp. Date_____

Signature_____

SEND ORDER TO: B.F. Publishing
                     P.O. Box 2712-344
                     Huntington Beach, CA 92647
                     800-544-7264

I Have a Choice?!
Order form to share with your friends.

☐ **YES,** rush my order for ____ copy(ies) of *I Have A Choice?!*
☐ to me, or ☐ send as a gift to a friend.
Book $12.95 ea. $_____

☐ **YES,** I want to take advantage of the new subscription rate for your newsletter informing me about new and alternative approaches to healing. I understand that if I am not completely satisfied, I can get a full refund within the first 90 days of my subscription.
One-Year Subscription $15.00 $_____

☐ **YES,** I firmly believe that education is the key to preventing dis-ease and dis-harmony, and that when the body is in balance, it is healthy. I want to help continue your commitment to disseminate educational information, create public awareness in the area of natural healing and promote research to find new and alternative approaches to healing.
Enclosed is my pledge of $_____

Add $4.00 S&H per book order $_____

CA residence add 7.75% sales tax $_____

TOTAL AMOUNT DUE $_____

Name_____

Street Address_____
(No P.O. Box Address)

City _____ State _____ Zip _____

Daytime Phone ( ) _____
(In case we have a question about your order.)

Payment Method:
☐ Check or money order payable to B.F. Publishing.
☐ Charge my ☐ MasterCard ☐ VISA ☐ Amex

Card # _____ Exp. Date_____

Signature_____

SEND ORDER TO: B.F. Publishing
P.O. Box 2712-344
Huntington Beach, CA 92647
800-544-7264

I Have a Choice?!

Order form to share with your friends.

☐ **YES,** rush my order for ____ copy(ies) of *I Have A Choice?!*
　　　　☐ to me, or ☐ send as a gift to a friend.

　　　　　　　　　　　　　　Book $12.95 ea. $_____

☐ **YES,** I want to take advantage of the new subscription rate for your newsletter informing me about new and alternative approaches to healing. I understand that if I am not completely satisfied, I can get a full refund within the first 90 days of my subscription.

　　　　　　　　　　　One-Year Subscription $15.00 $_____

☐ **YES,** I firmly believe that education is the key to preventing dis-ease and dis-harmony, and that when the body is in balance, it is healthy. I want to help continue your commitment to disseminate educational information, create public awareness in the area of natural healing and promote research to find new and alternative approaches to healing.

　　　　　　　　　　　Enclosed is my pledge of $_____

　　　　　　　　　　Add $4.00 S&H per book order $_____

　　　　　　　　　CA residence add 7.75% sales tax $_____

　　　　　　　　　　　　TOTAL AMOUNT DUE $_____

Name _____

Street Address _____
　　　　　　(No P.O. Box Address)

City _____ State _____ Zip _____

Daytime Phone (____) _____
　　　　　　　　(In case we have a question about your order.)

Payment Method:

☐ Check or money order payable to B.F. Publishing.

☐ Charge my　☐ MasterCard　☐ VISA　☐ Amex

Card # _____ Exp. Date _____

Signature _____

　　　　SEND ORDER TO:　B.F. Publishing
　　　　　　　　　　　　　　P.O. Box 2712-344
　　　　　　　　　　　　　　Huntington Beach, CA 92647
　　　　　　　　　　　　　　800-544-7264

I Have a Choice?!

Order form to share with your friends.

☐ **YES,** rush my order for _____ copy(ies) of *I Have A Choice?!*
  ☐ to me, or ☐ send as a gift to a friend.

  Book $12.95 ea. $_____

☐ **YES,** I want to take advantage of the new subscription rate for your newsletter informing me about new and alternative approaches to healing. I understand that if I am not completely satisfied, I can get a full refund within the first 90 days of my subscription.

  One-Year Subscription $15.00 $_____

☐ **YES,** I firmly believe that education is the key to preventing dis-ease and dis-harmony, and that when the body is in balance, it is healthy. I want to help continue your commitment to disseminate educational information, create public awareness in the area of natural healing and promote research to find new and alternative approaches to healing.

  Enclosed is my pledge of $_____

  Add $4.00 S&H per book order $_____

  CA residence add 7.75% sales tax $_____

  TOTAL AMOUNT DUE $_____

Name_____

Street Address_____
  (No P.O. Box Address)

City _____ State _____ Zip _____

Daytime Phone ( ) _____
  (In case we have a question about your order.)

Payment Method:

☐ Check or money order payable to B.F. Publishing.

☐ Charge my ☐ MasterCard ☐ VISA ☐ Amex

Card # _____ Exp. Date_____

Signature_____

SEND ORDER TO: B.F. Publishing
P.O. Box 2712-344
Huntington Beach, CA 92647
800-544-7264